# Simulation-Based Education

## A PRACTICAL APPROACH FOR HEALTH AND CARE EDUCATORS

*Edited by*

**ELIZABETH SIMPSON**

*Lecturer*
*Nursing & Health Care School*
*University of Glasgow*
*Glasgow, Scotland, UK*

**CLAIRE McGUINNESS**

*Professional Advisor, Nursing and Midwifery Education*
*Chief Nursing Officer's Directorate, Scottish Government*
*(Whilst editing this work, seconded from the substantive Post of Assistant Head Learning*
  *Teaching Quality, School of Health and Life Sciences, Glasgow Caledonian University)*

**CATIE PATON**

*Associate Director Medical Education*
*Clinical Skills Consultant*
*NHS Lanarkshire*
*Scotland, UK*

ELSEVIER

ISBN: 978-0-7020-8207-8

*Content Strategist:* Robert Edwards
*Content Project Manager:* Taranpreet Kaur
*Design:* Christian Bilbow
*Marketing Manager:* Deborah Watkins

Printed in India

Last digit is the print number: 9 8 7 6 5 4 3 2 1

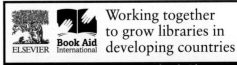

# PREFACE

S imulation education is historical in context, with evidence of its use and application in military exercises and, more recently, as part of aviation, medical and nursing and midwifery education. In the health and care context, simulation is now recognised as optimal for enabling and supporting learners to practice in a safe physical and psychological environment. This was perhaps more recently emphasised with the advent of the Covid-19 pandemic when health and care learners and educators were able to continue learning and teaching using a variety of simulation methods and approaches.

This book has harnessed the knowledge, skills, and expertise of a variety of health and care professionals with a vested interest in the development of simulation-based education (SBE). Consequently, the structure and content of this book have been designed to enable the reader to follow the journey of developing SBE. The journey represented as part of this book follows a logical and sequential approach to all components of SBE.

Furthermore, the ethos of the book is the provision of a 'workshop' in your pocket. That is to say, engaging with the content should be thought-provoking as well as instructional, enabling deep rather than surface learning. It has also been designed to enable the reader to select particular aspects to review and apply as appropriate, depending on the educational context and the needs of the learners. It is our hope that this book will not only demystify SBE but will demonstrate that SBE can be as simple or as complex as the presenting learning need demands.

Both novice and experienced educators experience challenges when attempting to engage with and develop simulation-based education (SBE). Whilst many SBE-focused texts exist, this book was commissioned with the intent of demonstrating that SBE need not be complex, labour-intensive, or expensive. It was also the aim to provide a stepwise approach to the development of each aspect of SBE, demonstrating the logic and applicability of this approach to learning and teaching across health and care professions. The contributors were selected on the basis of their expertise and knowledge of health and care and SBE, helping to ensure the engaging and practical nature of the book's content.

ELIZABETH SIMPSON, CLAIRE MCGUINNESS
AND CATIE PATON

# ACKNOWLEDGEMENTS

We would like to acknowledge the health and care professionals who supported the chapter contributors and editors in the creation of this book. Many thanks to Dr Ben Parkinson, Senior Lecturer and Chair of the Ethics Committee, School of Health and Life Sciences, Glasgow Caledonian University, for his time and expertise when reviewing the ethics content of Chapter 9.

ELIZABETH SIMPSON, CLAIRE McGUINNESS
AND CATIE PATON

*"It always seems impossible until it is done"*

**- NELSON MANDELA**

*This book is dedicated to all health and care professionals who have come to appreciate that education has the power to enable the achievement of the impossible.*

# CONTENTS

# CONTRIBUTORS

**ANDREA BAKER**
Skills and Simulation Manager
NHS Education for Scotland
Dundee, Scotland, UK

**FIONA BURTON**
Undergraduate Simulation Lead
University of Glasgow Medical School Consultant
    Emergency Medicine & Major Trauma
Queen Elizabeth University Hospital
Greater Glasgow & Clyde, UK

**KEITH CAMERON**
Advanced Paramedic

**VERONICA O'CARROLL**
Senior Lecturer
School of Medicine, University of St Andrews
St Andrews, Scotland, UK

**SHARON DONAGHY**
Senior Clinical Skills Specialist
Medical Education
NHS Lanarkshire

**NICHOLAS HOLT**
Consultant Physician Acute and General Medicine
University Hospital Monklands
Airdrie, NHS Lanarkshire

**ZOE HUTCHESON**
Emergency Medicine Specialty Doctor
NHS Lanarkshire
University Hospital Hairmyres
Scotland, UK
NHS Lanarkshire

**RONA KEAY**
Scottish Centre for Simulation and
    Clinical Human Factors
NHS Forth Valley

**DANIEL LYNAGH**
Specialist Registrar, Acute Internal Medicine
NHS GGC, Scotland
Honorary Clinical Lecturer
University of Glasgow
Glasgow, Scotland, UK

**GAYLE CAMPBELL MACKIE**
Campaign Manager
British Medical Association
Edinburgh, Scotland, UK

**CAROLINE MARTIN**
Senior Clinical Skills Specialist
Medical Education
NHS Lanarkshire

**ALISTAIR MAY**
Educational Coordinator
Scottish Centre for Simulation and Clinical Human
    Factors
NHS Forth Valley, Scotland, UK

**DAVID McARTHUR**
Lecturer (Digital Design)
Glasgow Caledonian University
Glasgow, Scotland, UK

**NEIL McGOWAN**
Associate Director Medical Education & Consultant
NHS Greater Glasgow and Clyde
Associate Professor
University of Glasgow
Glasgow, Scotland, UK

**CLAIRE McGUINNESS**
Professional Advisor, Nursing and Midwifery
   Education
Chief Nursing Officer's Directorate, Scottish
   Government
(Whilst editing this work, seconded from the
   substantive Post of Assistant Head Learning
   Teaching Quality, School of Health and Life
   Sciences, Glasgow Caledonian University)

**MAIRI McKINLEY**
Lead Clinical Educator
Department of Medical Education
NHS Fife
Kirkcaldy, Scotland, UK

**STEVEN MORRISON**
Watch Commander
Fire Safety Enforcement
City of Glasgow, Scottish Fire and Rescue Service
Glasgow, Scotland, UK

**JERRY MORSE**
Senior Lecturer in Clinical Simulation
Institute of Education in Healthcare and Medical
   Sciences
University of Aberdeen

**CATIE PATON**
Associate Director Medical Education
Clinical Skills Consultant
NHS Lanarkshire
Scotland, UK

**LINA PETRAKIEVA**
Academic Developer (Digital)
Glasgow Caledonian University
Glasgow, Scotland, UK

**KATH SHARP**
Head of Service - Physiotherapy, Children and Young
   People
NHS Lothian
Edinburgh, Scotland, UK

**ELIZABETH SIMPSON**
Lecturer
Nursing & Health Care School
University of Glasgow
Glasgow, Scotland, UK

**DICKSON NEILSON TELFER**
Learning Developer
Glasgow Caledonian University
Glasgow, Scotland, UK

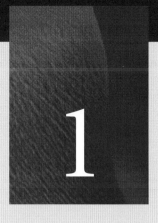

# 1

# INTRODUCTION TO SIMULATION-BASED EDUCATION IN HEALTH AND CARE

MAIRI McKINLEY ▪ VERONICA O'CARROLL

## CHAPTER OUTLINE

## OBJECTIVES

*This chapter should support the reader to develop an understanding of:*

- The historical development of simulation
- The importance of safety, and the role of human factors, in simulation-based education (SBE)
- Non-technical skills and technical skills
- The practicalities of the SBE teaching process
- The role of simulation in curricula
- Simulation in a pandemic
- The future of simulation

## KEY TERMS

Simulation

Human factors

Non-technical skills

Technical skills

Simulation-based education

SBE

Confederate

## INTRODUCTION

Simulation has become a key component of health and social care education. This book aims to provide a step-by-step guide to assist educators in the planning, implementation, and evaluation of simulation-based education (SBE) in health and social care. Central to this chapter is an overview of key components of SBE, alongside consideration of broader contemporary factors, including the recent COVID-19 pandemic, and the way in which this has impacted on the delivery of SBE for both learners and educators.

## BACKGROUND

Historically, simulation has been used in clinical education for many years. In fact, we know that early surgical simulators were in use more than 2500 years ago (Owen, 2012). Even then, these pioneers of simulation recognised the role simulators and anatomical models had in developing the confidence and competence of healthcare trainees and practitioners. Fast forward to the 21st century, SBE is no longer just about the use of simulators or manikins. In fact, simulation has been recognised as a technique to replace, augment, or amplify reality, rather than considered as a tool or a technology (Gaba, 2004).

Simulation has been further defined as 'a technique that creates a situation or environment to allow persons to experience a representation of a real event for the purpose of practice, learning, evaluation, testing, or to gain an understanding of systems or human actions' (Lioce et al., 2020, p. 44). From this definition, the move from considering simulation in healthcare as purely an educational tool, to that of one that enables evaluation of systems, and the interaction of humans within a system, is key. Simulation has been used in other 'high-risk' industries including aviation, nuclear energy, and the military for many years. Within these areas, simulation is seen as a technique to 'plan, reduce risk and increase control' (Ziv et al., 2000, p. 490). Comparisons are often made between healthcare and these types of 'high-risk' industries due to the inherent risks and complexities common across these types of systems. In addition, healthcare providers, along with other 'high-risk' industries, are often seen as 'safety critical' or high-reliability organisations (HROs). HROs are 'organisations that work in situations that have the potential for large-scale risk and harm, but which manage to balance effectiveness, efficiency and safety. They also minimise errors through teamwork, awareness of potential risk and constant improvement' (The Health Foundation, 2011, p. 3). Therefore, in addition to providing a technique to recreate reality, simulation allows the creation of a realistic scenario without the potential risks associated with a 'real' situation or environment. This is particularly relevant in health and social care as it enables learners, trainees, and practitioners to apply knowledge and gain experience of practical skills and procedures, without putting patients at risk. Examples of this could include managing an acutely unwell patient or dealing with an emergency situation.

As with all education activities, evaluating the outcomes of SBE is important, whether measuring the impact on learners or impact on their practice. While some uniprofessional and interprofessional evidence exists to support a positive impact on team performance and patient outcomes, the quality of this research is considered limited (Fransen et al., 2020; Marion-Martins and Pinho, 2020; Khan et al., 2018). Similarly, the longitudinal impact of preregistration SBE on post-registration practice is yet to be determined (Shiner, 2018). When considered in the context of the historical development of SBE, it is important to understand this, and to recognise that further research is required to gain a greater understanding of any potential impact.

## CONTEXT

### Safety and Simulation

We know that simulation is a technique which enables learners to develop their knowledge, skills, and confidence in a realistic environment, through immersion and experiential learning. The simulation activity will represent actual or potential real-world situations encountered in the learners' work environment. This can vary from everyday activities to potential hypothetical events, such as dealing with a major incident. The range of activities can be wide and can include everything from learning a new practical skill, to participating in a communication exercise. Communication exercises can range from those with a simulated patient, or with an embedded professional (faculty member with an embedded role within the scenario) adopting the role of a patient, relative, or health and social care professional, for a specific purpose aligned to the intended learning outcomes (ILOs) (Sanko et al., 2013). Often, simulation is described in relation to its fidelity, usually on a continuum of levels spanning low, medium, and high. Fidelity is defined as 'The degree to which the simulation replicates the real event and/or workplace; this includes physical, psychological, and environmental elements' (Lioce et al., 2020, p. 18). However, a high degree of fidelity is not necessarily required for an SBE activity to be successful, as this depends on many factors, including the level of experience of the learner in a particular environment, and the intended learning ILOs of the session. Table 1.1 identifies the different dimensions of fidelity that should be considered when designing an SBE activity. Consideration of each of these different dimensions will enable you to align the activity with the required ILOs.

| TABLE 1.1 | |
|---|---|
| **Dimensions of Fidelity** | |
| **Fidelity** | **Factors to Consider** |
| *Physical (or environmental)*<br>Determines the extent to which the physical context of the simulation-based activity replicates the actual 'real life' environment. | Simulated/standardised patient(s)<br>Use of a simulator/manikin<br>Environment: an adapted classroom, dedicated simulation lab/room, in-situ (actual) environment<br>Equipment/related props – real and/or simulated<br>presence of others/observers |
| *Conceptual*<br>Ensures that the different elements of the scenario or case are realistic and relate to each other, e.g., the history of the presenting complaint is consistent with the clinical findings. | Subject matter experts should be involved in the design/development of the case/scenario. The activity should be 'piloted' prior to being undertaken with learners. |
| *Psychological*<br>Endeavours to replicate the contextual aspects of the 'real' environment.<br>This component works synergistically with physical and conceptual fidelity to enhance learner engagement. | The provision of an 'active' voice for the patient/service user to enable realistic conversation to take place.<br>Factors inherent to the 'real' environment such as lighting and noise, distractions, the presence of 'actors' playing the parts of family members and/or healthcare team members.<br>The inclusion of time-restricted deadlines, competing priorities. |

Modified from INACSL Standards Committee, 2016.

SBE may take many forms, ranging from simulated, virtual patients, or virtual relatives, part-task trainers, interactive and non-interactive manikins, screen-based (computer) simulations, and gaming (Aggarwal et al., 2010). However, the extent to which each of these approaches is used will be influenced by a number of factors including the ILOs, time available, access to facilities, resources (including equipment and consumables), simulated patients, all faculty, and the finances available to procure, maintain, and replace equipment and software. The use of some of these different approaches will be discussed in more detail in Chapter 5 when considering the use of SBE for skill acquisition.

A carefully planned and delivered SBE session has the potential to provide a physically and psychologically safe learning environment. This enables the practice of both technical skills (TS) and non-technical skills (NTS) without risk of harm to real patients, as well as reducing the stress and anxiety experienced by learners, when compared to the real clinical environment (Dearmon et al., 2016). Therefore, when designing simulations, we must strive to create an authentic learning experience within a realistic but non-threatening environment (Al-Ghareeb and Cooper, 2016). By creating such an environment, SBE provides a powerful tool to assist learners in the transfer of theoretical knowledge to practical application or, in other words, bridging the theory–practice gap. In support of this, there is growing evidence that employing SBE as a technique in healthcare education improves learners' knowledge, skills, and confidence levels (Alanazi et al., 2017).

Patient safety is crucial and is defined as actions undertaken by individuals and organisations to protect healthcare recipients from being harmed by their healthcare (The National Patient Safety Association, 2008). In 2000, in their seminal report '*To err is human*', the Institute of Medicine (IoM) recommended that SBE should be used as a key strategy for reducing avoidable harm in healthcare (IoM, 2000). We know SBE features significantly in many healthcare students' curricula (Cant and Cooper, 2017) and the importance of simulation is emphasised as an integral part of patient safety curricula by the World Health Organization (WHO, 2011).

There is growing evidence that health and social care SBE contributes to improved quality of care and survival through skills and teams training (Donoghue et al., 2021). Aligning with this, an international group of researchers and experts in simulation identified five main areas for consideration when adopting SBE within patient safety–focused curricula (Sollid et al., 2019). These are:

1. Non-technical skills (NTS)
2. Technical skills (TS)
3. System probing
4. Assessment
5. Effectiveness

Currently there is more evidence available relating to the first three areas, with assessment and effectiveness of simulation, and the impact of these on patient safety, requiring further research (Sollid et al., 2019).

## Human Factors

Human factors is a science incorporated as part of education by several industries, particularly the high-risk professions including aviation, aerospace, and the military. This term describes the environmental, organisational and occupational factors, and the human elements, that impact on behaviours and can ultimately affect safety (Health and Safety Executive, 2022). Understanding human factors allows organisations to optimise human performance, enabling people to be more efficient, safer, and reliable. Accepting that the human condition cannot be changed, and acknowledging human limitations, means looking to other factors, and changing the conditions under which humans operate. This will allow minimising of, and mitigation for, frailties, risk, and reduction of error.

Human factors training merges powerfully with SBE for Interprofessional Learning (IPL). Simulation can be purposefully stressful in design to replicate reality and to challenge the learner in a safe and supportive environment. This provides an opportunity for learners and teams to reflect on the effects of stress, and its impact on cognitive load and NTS. It also enables interprofessional teams to experience and prepare for the management of critical incidents that normally occur less frequently. This can improve team working, communication, and leadership (Siassakos et al., 2011). (Refer to Chapters 3 and 5 for additional information on human factors and NTS.)

## AN OVERVIEW OF MASTERY-BASED LEARNING

Mastery-based learning is an educational approach originating in work first described by John Carroll, a Professor of Educational Psychology at Harvard University, during the early 1960s (Carroll, 1963). The approach is based on two beliefs:

1. All learners can (and will) uniformly achieve a performance goal or task completion.
2. Some learners will take longer than others to achieve the performance goal.

This therefore indicates that given enough time, all learners will achieve a similar level of proficiency, through a competency-based learning approach, in a procedure or skill. This is more evident when the learner is highly motivated. Mastery learning is a very stringent form of competency-based education which has overlapping elements associated with deliberate practice. It has nine key complementary features (McGaghie et al., 2010):

1. Highly motivated learners, with good concentration, who address
2. Well-defined learning objectives or tasks at an
3. Appropriate level of difficulty, with
4. Focused, repetitive practice that yields
5. Rigorous, reliable measurements, that provide
6. Informative feedback from educational sources (e.g., simulators, teachers), that promotes
7. Monitoring, error correction, and more deliberate practice, that enables
8. Evaluation and performance that may reach a mastery standard, where learning time may vary but expected minimal outcomes are identical, and allows
9. Advancement to the next task or unit.

These nine features ensure that all learners accomplish learning with little or no variation in the agreed standard (McGaghie et al., 2010). However, there may be variation in the time taken to achieve the necessary level of performance, which could be considered problematic by some educators. Nevertheless, there is a growing body of evidence around simulation-based mastery learning (SBML) demonstrating the direct impact SBML programmes have in improving patient outcomes, particularly in relation to high-risk procedures (e.g., tracheal intubation or lumbar puncture) (Barsuk et al., 2018; McGaghie et al., 2014). Similarly, SBML has been shown to improve the competence and confidence of healthcare professionals (Scahill et al., 2021) which has led to improvements in the quality of healthcare delivered, and reduced risk of iatrogenic harm. As a result, educators have continued to develop SBML programs in many different areas of health and social care, including high-risk procedural skills as well as programs to improve complex communication skills (Vermylen et al., 2019).

The disadvantage of SBML is that this can be a resource intensive teaching and learning strategy. To address this some educators have adapted their programmes and include pre-learning and peer learning activities (Scahill et al., 2021). These adaptations appear to be very promising in enabling SBML programs to be delivered, but in a less resource-intense way (Scahill et al., 2021).

## DEFINING SKILLS

Historically skills in healthcare were taught using an apprenticeship style approach of *see one, do one, teach one*, where learners initially observed a task, then practised the task (usually only once), before then being expected to teach the task to another learner. This practice did not account for different learning styles, learner dexterity or ability and, at times, it could be argued that practice may not have been evidence-based. Simulation enables the opportunity to move away from the 'see one do one teach one' (Rodriguez-Paz et al., 2009) approach to developing skills, to a space where the individual is supported to develop skills at their own pace. By creating an authentic, safe, patient-free environment learners can practice both TS and NTS with constructive feedback, enabling the learner to grow in competence and confidence in this safe environment. This experience enhances patient safety as learners have practiced and accomplished the required skills prior to direct patient contact.

### Non-technical Skills

NTS are defined as 'the cognitive, social and personal resource skills that complement TS and contribute to safe and efficient task performance' (Flin et al., 2008, p. 1). Key NTS that have been identified as important within the healthcare environment include:

- **Social skills,** such as communication, teamwork, and leadership

- **Cognitive skills,** such as decision making and situational awareness
- **Personal resource skills,** such as how an individual manages stress and copes with fatigue.

Initially, the work around using SBE to improve non-TS in health and social care focused primarily on staff working in operating theatres (Flin, 2013); however, this is now found in most areas of health and social care including emergency departments, clinics, and wards (Hull and Sevdalis, 2015). SBE can be used to develop effective NTS for the individual health and social care professional or team and has been shown to be a more effective learning and teaching strategy than didactic methods (Griffin et al., 2019). An example of this is given by Kaplonyi et al. (2017) who found using role play with simulated patients or health and social care professionals was effective in allowing practise of communication skills between these professionals, patients, and their families. The outcome of this was improved patient satisfaction and safer health and social care overall. More recently, several tools have been validated to assess both the individual's and team's NTS (Ounounou et al., 2019).

### Technical Skills

Within the health and social care context, TS are normally procedural and involve the development of ability through practice and repetition, alongside constructive feedback. Simulation can be used as a strategy to build learners' confidence and ability in TS. By creating a non-threatening environment, where learners have the opportunity for multiple attempts to practise, constructive feedback can be provided, contributing to the development of these TS. This development of skills can be greatly enhanced using the principles associated with mastery learning. In addition to providing the opportunity to practice skills and procedures, SBE has also been shown to improve the confidence of trainees to manage similar real-life scenarios (Hecimovich and Volet, 2011).

## THE TEACHING PROCESS IN SIMULATION

Throughout this book, reference will be made to the planning, briefing, delivery, and debriefing elements of the SBE teaching process. We will now consider these elements which are essential in the facilitation of TS and NTS acquisition.

## Planning

This is the first step of the teaching process and consideration of several elements of this is required, including:

- Why has simulation been chosen?
- What is/are the intended learning objective(s)?
- Who are the faculty and what contribution can they make?
- Where and when will the simulation activity take place?
- Who are the learners and what are their needs (learning outcomes)?
- How will the experience be evaluated?

In light of this, it is essential, at the earliest opportunity, to share timelines and expectations of everyone involved in the development of the educational event. This information will also guide the development of the scenario(s) which will help to structure the event.

## Briefing

Briefing is key to the success of the simulation and the faculty delivering the session must clearly outline the session plan. This means both faculty and learners should be aware of their roles and responsibilities throughout the session, and an agenda should be set based on their individual expectations and session ILOs. This will help to ensure that everyone is in agreement and therefore has a shared mental model moving forward (Konnings et al., 2021).

### Faculty Briefing

A meeting with faculty should be planned to take place prior to the arrival of learners. It is good practice to prepare briefing notes and a checklist relating to the simulation session in advance of this meeting, frequently referred to as a faculty briefing. This sets the scene for faculty, allowing for discussion where faculty can highlight areas of concern or queries. While this is of value for all simulation sessions, it is of particular benefit when delivering sessions to a large cohort of learners with large faculty numbers. This approach will aid standardisation of the delivery and will also promote an equitable learner experience, irrespective of which faculty member(s) are delivering. It is also an opportunity to discuss sensitive information regarding learners which may impact on, or influence, the learners' experience. For example, a learner may disclose details which require reasonable adjustments to the session. This could include a learner with dyslexia, who requires a coloured, transparent overlay to allow them to read documents.

### Learner Briefing

The learners' briefing should set the scene for the session and outline the session plan. It is important to review the timetable or schedule with the learners, including informing them of planned breaktimes. This may seem a trivial point, but this level of detail demonstrates you have considered learners' needs and are sensitive to these, which can help alleviate any anxieties they may be experiencing.

Ground rules for the session should be set in partnership with learners. While the teaching and learning environment should be supportive, and to some extent relaxed to engage the learner, expectations regarding professionalism and behaviours should be discussed and agreed with learners in advance. An integral feature of any ground rules should be respect for colleagues and maintenance of confidentiality. This promotes a trusting learning environment in which learners genuinely are free to make mistakes without consequence. Together, these lay the foundation for psychological safety of learners throughout the simulation. Some simulation centres use cameras for feedback purposes in the debrief, and learners are normally advised of this in advance to ensure they are aware of this before they attend. Nevertheless, the thought of being filmed can be a source of anxiety for some learners. To help alleviate anxiety, facilitators must disclose the ways in which cameras will be used for learning, the limitations of access to the recordings and confirmation of permission from the learners. Any other use of recordings, for example for conference presentations or faculty development courses, will require additional written consent from learners. As the purposes of using recordings in these situations are not integral to the learning experience, learners can refuse, and this must be respected.

With the scene set, ground rules and professional expectations agreed, the briefing session should then move on to reviewing the ILOs for the session and exploring the learners' personal objectives to establish what they would like to achieve during the session. This gives learners ownership of their own learning and generates partnership working. Learners' personal objectives should be invited by the facilitator and shared and written on the board, at the outset of the session. The purpose of doing this is to allow the facilitator to return to these at the end of the session to evaluate if the planned ILOs *and* learners' personal objectives have been met.

The briefing session is an ideal opportunity to introduce learners to the technology and equipment they will be using during the session. Here learners can become familiar with the functionality and capabilities of manikins, skills trainers, monitoring equipment, and consumables being used. By doing this, the focus of the session can be on the skill or scenario and the authenticity of the session will be enhanced. Furthermore, the debriefing session is more likely to generate discussion around the planned ILOs, rather than being monopolised by challenges faced due to lack of familiarity with equipment.

### Delivery

While the nature of the simulation event itself may vary from a table-top exercise to clinical skill or a scenario-based approach, the principles of the delivery are similar across all. From a learner's perspective this may be considered the main event; however, for the facilitator, this is where we begin the execution of our teaching plan. We need to create an environment which is authentic, safe for learners to make mistakes and allows them to apply the evidence base to their practice.

Delivery of the session involves direct contact with the learners, encouraging them to become immersed and engaged in the simulation. Student engagement has been defined as 'the product of motivation and active learning. It is a product rather than a sum because it will not occur if either elements are missing' (Barkley, 2010, p. 6). Participation during the delivery of a simulation can account for Barkley's (2010) *active element*, and as facilitators of simulation we must *motivate* learners by the creation of a positive learning environment.

### Debriefing

Debriefing is pivotal in the process of learning in SBE, and selection of an appropriate debriefing framework is key. The debriefing strategy should be agreed at the faculty briefing. Single debriefing by one facilitator or co-debriefing by two or more facilitators should be discussed to clarify roles to ensure the smooth delivery of the session. There are different techniques which can be adopted to generate discussion among learners during the debrief. Examples of these include advocacy with inquiry or a learning conversation. The advocacy with inquiry technique seeks to explore the learner's thought processes that influenced their behaviour, whereas the learning conversation supports reflective discussion. Both have the aim of generating new knowledge to improve future practice. It is important to plan which model of debriefing will be used, as there are many. Debriefing models will further explored in Chapter 3.

## SIMULATION-BASED EDUCATION AND THE COVID-19 PANDEMIC

Although some guidance existed for health and social care organisations to prepare for public health emergencies (WHO, 2017), guidance for the broader use of simulation in health and social care education continues to be limited. This reinforces the need for educators in these fields to carefully consider the planning and implementation of SBE. This became even more apparent during the COVID-19 pandemic which manifested towards the end of 2019. Aspects including delivery, level of learner, creation of resources, and appropriate measurement of learning outcomes (LOs) to determine the impact of SBE, became even more important during the pandemic as simulation was prioritised as a key authentic substitution for direct patient-contact practice learning.

### Health and Social Care Education

During the COVID-19 pandemic, educators were faced with the reality that, for this period at least, health and social care delivery had to take precedence over facilitating learning for students in practice placements. Educators were faced with the predicament of ensuring that final year undergraduates, sometimes referred to as pre-qualifying students, could achieve the required learning before professional registration. To relieve pressure on practice placement providers, professional governing bodies, in some countries, endorsed simulation as an acceptable alternative for healthcare students to gain practical experience. However, guidance on the implementation of SBE to achieve this varied between governing bodies and ranged from clear, specific guidance to none at all. Some professional governing bodies stipulated a maximum number of hours over the duration of a programme (Nursing and Midwifery Council (NMC), 2021), while others placed the emphasis on the quality of the SBE experience. Overall, the need for high quality, robust, reliable, and replicable SBE was recognised (Health and Care Professions Council (HCPC), 2021). Clear and collaborative dialogue between professional bodies and universities was key to the implementation of SBE as a substitute for practice learning. This collaboration was to ensure all parties satisfaction with the planned alternative approach. Universities responsible for the delivery of health and social care education had to liaise closely with practice partners to develop SBE that was authentic and closely aligned with real-life practice learning experiences. The pace at which this change took place meant a challenging time for all involved as this also coincided with the large-scale move to digital learning. This was essential to ensure the continuation of education for learners who would ultimately contribute to the delivery of care during this unprecedented global event.

## Practice Learning

Despite the pressures on resources within health and social care during the pandemic, SBE was valued and prioritised as a necessary and vital measure to ensure that health and social care workers were adequately prepared for the delivery of safe and effective care. Within practice settings, SBE became a vehicle to support the upskilling of staff, who were redeployed to new and unfamiliar roles in response to the pandemic (Pan and Rajwani, 2021). Similarly, structured, evidence-based simulation played an important role in anaesthesia, where it was contextualised to practise the additional measures required when treating patients with COVID-19, including donning and doffing of personal protective equipment (PPE) and airway management skills. At the height of the pandemic, in-situ and laboratory-based SBE was used to develop health and social care workers' TS and NTS. It was reported that this had a positive influence on both the mental preparedness and assertiveness of practitioners during teamwork (Cheung et al., 2020).

## THE FUTURE OF SIMULATION-BASED EDUCATION

Innovations in digital technology, including extended reality SBE, provide opportunities for remote learning and helps to link educators and learners globally. Extended reality, which encompasses virtual reality (VR), augmented reality (AR), and mixed reality (MR), has now been proven to impact significantly on educational and health and social care outcomes.

VR immerses the learner in a complete virtual experience, replacing what the person sees and experiences. Sensory equipment enables digital interaction with the virtual world. VR-based surgical simulation has been used and there is evidence to confirm the positive impact on skill performance and improved patient outcomes (Aghazadeh et al., 2016; Gerull et al., 2020). This technology is being pushed further to explore the use of haptics (sense of touch) as a feedback tool. However, it is likely to be some time before the true impact of VR on practice is demonstrated, and before it becomes accessible in terms of cost (Rangarajan et al., 2020).

AR combines the physical and virtual environment. It uses a real-time combination of a physical setting augmented by virtual imagery, through devices such as smart glasses or projection technologies. Some AR technology is portable and can be used outside of specific educational setting such as a laboratory or skills centres. The benefit of portable or mobile AR is the accessibility it offers, which can make learning available to health and social care professionals within real health and social care settings. This is important for continuing professional development and may add another dimension to simulation within health and social care settings. AR has been used extensively in surgical training and its use beyond this is increasingly being explored. Tang et al. (2020) report that, to date, AR has been used across a range of specialities from acquisition of a clinical skill (e.g., suturing) to the more complex procedural skills (e.g., laparoscopic cholecystectomy). Once again, further high-quality research is required to build on the evidence to demonstrate its impact on practice (Gerup et al. 2020; Tang et al., 2020).

MR combines elements of virtual and augmented reality, allowing real-world interaction with virtual data, in real time. MR is used in SBE and also in real practice, an example of which includes the use of virtual data used during surgical practice (Cartucho et al., 2020).

Learning technology is constantly evolving and opening up new opportunities to enable the delivery and assessment of high-quality remote SBE. This software is far more accessible and flexible for learners and educators than ever before, without the need for expensive equipment. For example, mobile phone applications can be used to record for in-situ simulation and, as part of this, recordings can be shared securely for group debriefs involving remote learners. This, and other aspects of technology-enhanced learning, will be discussed as part of Chapter 2.

With increased use of telehealth and telecare, simulation may improve health and social care staff confidence and their ability to engage effectively with this technology. Furthermore, it can help prepare undergraduate students in the use of digital tools in their practice. SBE using telehealth scenarios may lend themselves well to the remote learning environment. Learners can connect with standardised or real patients to work through a teleconsultation. From an interprofessional learning perspective, there is the opportunity to explore the use of telehealth for interprofessional collaboration between remotely located teams.

## TOP TIPS

Now that we have introduced you to the concept of SBE, here are a few tips to consider and reflect upon before moving on to Chapter 2:

| Top Tip | Guidance |
| --- | --- |
| ■ **Work with those who challenge and inspire you** | When setting up a simulation-based education (SBE) initiative, working with people who have the same goal and have the same passion for a quality learning experience is important. However, it is important to open your mind to new ideas and perspectives. Particularly in the planning stages of an SBE initiative, bringing in a variety of opinions and perspectives will encourage creativity and better problem solving. |

| Top Tip | Guidance |
| --- | --- |
| ■ **Do not reinvent what has already been invented** | The path of SBE is well trodden, and new paths are being created continually. Networking with other organisations that have experience of what you are trying to achieve is a great way to learn from others (the good, the bad, and the ugly) and will save time in the long run. People generally like talking about what they have achieved and will be willing to share. Seek advice from people in seminars or conferences. Consult the literature; educational journals in the field of healthcare education often publish short reports related to SBE initiatives that are a work in progress or have been implemented and evaluated. This is also a good way to find pretested, validated tools that can be used to measure the impact of your SBE. |
| ■ **Remember that simulation does not have to be expensive** | The equipment and technology now available is wide-ranging and new innovations are constantly being developed. However, regardless of the equipment that is used, and how advanced or fundamental it is, the main principles for effective SBE are the same. Effective SBE can be achieved with minimal equipment and some imagination. |
| ■ **Think about the fundamentals first** | The fundamental underpinning educational principles used in planning and designing any SBE initiative will always apply. Take the time to think about these before beginning: ■ Who are the learners? ■ What are the intended learning outcomes (ILOs)? ■ How can the learning be evaluated? |

| Top Tip | Guidance | Top Tip | Guidance |
|---------|----------|---------|----------|
| ■ **Recognise that you cannot do it all** | You have come up with a great SBE idea, you are highly motivated to make it work, but you may well feel obligated to see the journey through single-handedly, without feeling you are burdening others. Let others provide support and do not be afraid to ask for help. Use their skills and seek out the expertise around you. Your motivation, energy, and vision will inspire others, and you will reach your goal through your teams' collaborative efforts. This is a much more rewarding, achievable, and sustainable way of achieving a quality SBE experience that you may even want to repeat again or indeed expand. | ■ **Stay with the script** | It may be necessary to adapt or interject to move the scenario along; however, straying from the script or scenario can be catastrophic and lead the simulation away from the aim and purpose of the session. Do not be tempted to kill the mannikin to create drama. This could lead to learners feeling confused and demoralised that they have not achieved the learning outcomes. |
| ■ **Pay attention to the detail** | The detail is important, particularly to help learners feel that this is an authentic SBE experience. Think of your simulation learning environment as a stage hosting a play. Think of the SBE scenario as a storyline or plot; the simulated patients and/or carers/relatives are the characters, the facilitator is the director, and the stagehands are the SBE technicians who will provide support for the moulage and the equipment. Rehearsing the scenario and mapping out key events on a timeline can be helpful preparation. Share this timeline with all faculty before the simulation. This can help to anticipate the 'next scene' as the simulation is in progress. | ■ **If it isn't broken, don't fix it** | Following a successful simulation, you and your team will feel energised and will want to do it all over again, but next time, bigger and better with even more bells and whistles. It is a natural and fantastic feeling. It is important to debrief with your team and reflect on what went well and what could be improved. You may decide to note some changes required for improvement, or to troubleshoot any obvious issues for the next time. However, only tweak if needed and be guided once again by the aim of the sessions and ILOs. |

| Top Tip | Guidance |
|---|---|
| ■ **Remember that all good things must come to an end** | Know when an SBE activity has run its course and may need to be redesigned, or possibly just needs to stop. Things to consider include:<br>■ Can the SBE activity be sustained over time?<br>■ Are new ILOs required as a consequence of curricula or service change?<br>■ Does the SBE activity continue to meet the LOs?<br>■ Does the SBE activity remain the best strategy for learning?<br>■ Is it time to develop something new?<br>■ Are you carrying forward your learning and achievements and using that energy for new developments? |
| ■ **Share your work** | It can be challenging to find the time to share your good SBE work, or maybe you feel that it is not worth sharing. However, sharing your knowledge and disseminating your work will help to build the evidence base for effective SBE. Healthcare education–focussed journals, conferences, and seminars often welcome short descriptive reports, initial findings from SBE evaluations, or lessons learned from a new SBE initiative. Remember this and consider sharing your good practice to contribute to the evidence base. |

## SUMMARY

*From little acorns, mighty oak trees grow.*
*(Anonymous)*

SBE is multifaceted and requires an understanding of the underlying principles and language associated with this educational approach. Knowing where and how to start can be challenging for anyone setting out to design and implement an SBE activity. This chapter has sought to present the fundamental concepts to start you on the journey of considering how this approach to learning and teaching can be implemented in your own environment. Remember, what may seem small and insignificant as a first idea can be the start of something bigger and better. Moving forward, this book will serve as a guide for those wishing to set off on the SBE journey and, more importantly, it should enable you to work collaboratively with faculty to design and plan high-quality SBE experiences for learners. It should also empower you to be innovative and creative in your role as simulation educator.

## REFERENCES

Aggarwal, R., Mytton, O.T., Derbrew, M., et al., 2010. Training and simulation for patient safety. BMJ Qual. Saf. 19, i34–i43.

Aghazadeh, M.A., Mercado, M.A., Pan, M.M., et al., 2016. Performance of robotic simulated skills tasks is positively associated with clinical robotic surgical performance. BJU Int. 118 (3), 475–481.

Alanazi, A.A., Nicholson, N., Thomas, S., 2017. The use of simulation training to improve knowledge, skills, and confidence among healthcare students: A systematic review. Internet J. Allied. Health Sci. Pract. 15 (3), Article 2.

Al-Ghareeb, A., Cooper, S.J., 2016. Barriers and enablers to the use of high-fidelity patient simulation manikins in nurse education: An integrative review. Nurse Educ. Today 36, 281–286. https://doi.org/10.1016/j.nedt.2015.08.005.

Barkley, E.F., 2010. Student Engagement Techniques: A Handbook for College Faculty. Jossey-Bass, San Francisco.

Barsuk, J.H., Cohen, E.R., Williams, M.V., et al., 2018. Simulation-based mastery learning for thoracentesis skills improves patient outcomes: A randomized trial. Acad. Med. 93 (5), 729–735. https://doi.org/10.1097/ACM.0000000000001965.

Cant, R.P., Cooper, S.J., 2017. Use of simulation-based learning in undergraduate nursing education: An umbrella systematic review. Nurse Educ. Today 49, 63–71. https://doi.org/10.1016/j.nedt.2016.11.015.

Carroll, J., 1963. A model of school learning. Teach Coll. Record. 64, 723–733. https://www.tcrecord.org/books/Content.asp?ContentID=2839. (Accessed 11 September 2021).

Cartucho, J., Shapira, D., Ashrafian, H., Giannarou, S., 2020. Multimodal mixed reality visualisation for intraoperative surgical guidance. Int. J. Comput. Assist. Radiol. Surg. 15 (5), 819–826.

Cheung, V.K., So, E.H., Ng, G.W., et al., 2020. Investigating effects of healthcare simulation on personal strengths and organizational impacts for healthcare workers during COVID-19 pandemic: a cross-sectional study. Integr. Med. Res. 9 (3):100476. https://doi.org/10.1016/j.imr.2020.100476.

Dearmon, V., Graves, R.J., Hayden, S., et al., 2012. Effectiveness of simulation-based orientation of baccalaureate nursing students preparing for their first clinical experience. J. Nurs. Educ. 52 (1), 29–38. https://doi.org/10.3928/01484834-20121212-02.

Donoghue, A., Navarro, K., Diederich, E., et al., 2021. Deliberate practice and mastery learning in resuscitation education: A scoping review. Resusc. Plus 15 (6),100137. https://doi.org/10.1016/j.resplu.2021.100137.

Flin, R., O'Connor, P., Crichton, M., 2008. Safety at the Sharp End: A Guide to Non-Technical Skills. Ashgate, Aldershot.

Flin, R., 2013. Non-Technical Skills for Anaesthetists, Surgeons and Scrub Practitioners (ANTS, NOTSS and SPLINTS). The Health Foundation, London. https://improve.bmj.com/sites/default/files/resources/non_technical_skills_for_anaesthetists_surgeons_and_scrub_practitioners.pdf. (Accessed 15 July 2021).

Fransen, A.F., van de Ven, J., Banga, F.R., et al., 2020. Multi-professional simulation-based team training in obstetric emergencies for improving patient outcomes and trainees' performance. Cochrane Database Syst. Rev. Issue 12. Art. No.: CD011545. https://doi.org/10.1002/14651858.CD011545.pub2.

Gaba, D.M., 2004. The future vision of simulation in health care. Qual. Saf. Health Care 13, 2–10. https://doi.org/10.1136/qshc.2004.009878.

Gerull, W., Zihni, A., Awad, M., 2020. Operative performance outcomes of a simulator-based robotic surgical skills curriculum. Surg. Endosc. 34 (10), 4543–4548.

Gerup, J., Soerensen, C.B., Dieckmann, P., 2020. Augmented reality and mixed reality for healthcare education beyond surgery: An integrative review. Int. J. Med. Educ. 11, 1–18. https://doi.org/10.5116/ijme.5e01.eb1a1.

Griffin, C., Aydın, A., Brunckhorst, O., et al., 2019. Non-technical skills: A review of training and evaluation in urology. World J. Urol. 4, 1–9.

Health and Safety Executive, 2022. Introduction to human factors. https://www.hse.gov.uk/humanfactors/introduction.htm. (Accessed 07 July 2023).

Health and Care Professions Council, 2021. Advice for education providers. https://www.hcpc-uk.org/covid-19/advice/advice-for-education-providers/. (Accessed 15 July 2021).

Health Foundation, 2011. High Reliability Organizations. The Health Foundation, London. https://www.health.org.uk/publications/high-reliability-organizations. (Accessed 2 August 2021).

Hecimovich, M., Volet, S., 2011. Development of professional confidence in health education: Research evidence of the impact of guided practice into the profession. Health Educ. 111 (3), 177–197.

Hull, L., Sevdalis, N., 2015. Advances in teaching and assessing nontechnical skills. Surg. Clin. N. Am. 95, 869–884. https://doi.org/10.1016/j.suc.2015.04.003.

Institute of Medicine, 2000. To Err Is Human: Building a Safer Health System. The National Academies Press, Washington, DC. https://doi.org/10.17226/9728.

International Nursing Association for Clinical Simulation and Learning (INACSL) Standards Committee, 2016. INACSL standards of best practice: Simulation[SM] simulation design. Clin. Simul. Nurs. 12 (S), S5–S12. 10.1016/ j.ecns.2016.09.005.

Kaplonyi, J., Bowles, K.A., Nestel, D., et al., 2017. Understanding the impact of simulated patients on health care learners' communication skills: A systematic review. Med. Educ. 51, 1209–1219.

Könings, K.D., Mordang, S., Smeenk, F., Stassen, L., Ramani, S., 2021. Learner involvement in the co-creation of teaching and learning: AMEE Guide No. 138. Medical Teacher 43 (8), 924–936. https://doi.org/10.1080/0142159X.2020.1838464.

Khan, R., Plahouras, J., Johnston, B.C., et al., 2018. Virtual reality simulation training for health professions trainees in gastrointestinal endoscopy. Cochrane Database Syst. Rev. Issue 8. Art. No.: CD008237. https://doi.org/10.1002/14651858.CD008237.pub3.

Lioce, L., Lopreiato, J., Downing, D., et al., 2020. Healthcare Simulation Dictionary, 2nd ed. Rockville, MD. Agency for Healthcare Research and Quality. https://doi.org/10.23970/simulationv2.

Marion-Martins, A.D., Pinho, D.L.M., 2020. Interprofessional simulation effects for healthcare students: A systematic review and meta-analysis. Nurse Educ. Today 94,104568. https://doi.org/10.1016/j.nedt.2020.104568.

McGaghie, W.C., Issenberg, S.B., Barsuk, J.H., et al., 2014. A critical review of simulation-based mastery learning with translational outcomes. Med. Educ. 48 (4), 375–385. https://doi.org/10.1111/medu.12391.

McGaghie, W.C., Issenberg, S.B., Petrusa, E.R., et al., 2010. A critical review of simulation-based medical education research: 2003–2009. Med. Educ. 44, 50–63. https://doi.org/10.1111/j.1365-2923.2009.03547.x.

National Patient Safety Foundation, 2008. The National Patient Safety Foundation. http://www.npsf.org/. (Accessed 21 August 2021).

Nursing and Midwifery Council, 2021. Current emergency and recovery programme standards. https://www.nmc.org.uk/globalassets/sitedocuments/education-standards/current-emergency-and-recovery-programme-standards.pdf. (Accessed 19 July 2021).

Ounounou, E., Aydin, A., Brunckhorst, O., et al., 2019. Nontechnical skills in surgery: A systematic review of current training modalities. J. Surg. Educ. 76, 14–24.

Owen, H., 2012. Early use of simulation in medical education. Simul. Healthc. 7 (2), 102–116. https://doi.org/10.1097/SIH.0b013e3182415a91.

Pan, D., Rajwani, K., 2021. Implementation of simulation training during the COVID-19 pandemic: A New York hospital experience. Simul. Healthc. 16 (1), 46–51. https://doi.org/10.1097/SIH.0000000000000535.

Rangarajan, K., Davis, H., Pucher, P.H., 2020. Systematic review of virtual haptics in surgical simulation: A valid educational tool? J. Surg. Educ. 77 (2), 337–347.

Rodriguez-Paz, J.M., Kennedy, M., Salas, E., et al., 2009. Beyond "see one, do one, teach one": Toward a different training paradigm. BMJ Quality & Safety 18, 63–68.

Sanko, J.S., Shekhter, I., Kyle Jr., R.R., et al., 2013. Establishing a convention for acting in healthcare simulation: Merging art and science. Simul. Healthc. 8 (4), 215–220.

Scahill, E.L., Oliver, N.G., Tallentire, V.R., et al., 2021. An enhanced approach to simulation-based mastery learning: Optimising the educational impact of a novel, National Postgraduate Medical Boot Camp. Adv. Simul. 6, 15. https://doi.org/10.1186/s41077-021-00157-1.

Shiner, N., 2018. Is there a role for simulation-based education within conventional diagnostic radiography? A literature review. Radiography 24 (3), 262–271. https://doi.org/10.1016/j.radi.2018.01.006.

Siassakos, D., Bristowe, K., Hambly, H., Angouri, J., Crofts, J.F., Winter, C., Hunt, L.P., Draycott, T.J. 2011. Team communication with patient actors: findings from a multisite simulation study. Simul Healthc. 6 (3), 143–9. https://doi.org/10.1097/SIH.0b013e31821687cf.

Sollid, S.J.M., Dieckman, P., Aase, K., et al., 2019. Five topics health care simulation can address to improve patient safety: Results from a consensus process. J. Patient Saf. 15 (2), 111–120. https://doi.org/10.1097/PTS.0000000000000254.

Tang, K.S., Cheng, D.L., Mi, E., Greenberg, P.B., 2020. Augmented reality in medical education: A systematic review. Can. Med. Educ. J. 11 (1), e81–e96. https://doi.org/10.36834/cmej.61705.

Vermylen, J.H., Wood, G.J., Cohen, E.R., Barsuk, J.H., McGaghie, W.C., Wayne, D.B., 2019. Development of a simulation-based mastery learning curriculum for breaking bad news. J. Pain Symptom Manage 57 (3), 682–687. https://doi.org/10.1016/j.jpainsymman.2018.11.012.

World Health Organization, 2011. Patient Safety Curriculum Guide: Multi-professional Edition. WHO Press, Geneva.

World Health Organization, 2017. WHO simulation exercise manual: A practical guide and tool for planning, conducting and evaluating simulation exercises for outbreaks and public health emergency preparedness and response. WHO Press, Geneva. https://apps.who.int/iris/handle/10665/254741.

Ziv, A., Small, S.D., Wolpe, P.R., 2000. Patient safety and simulation-based medical education. Med. Teach. 22 (5), 489–495.

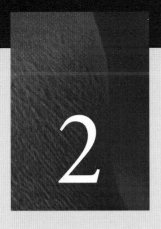

2

# INTERACTIVE REUSABLE LEARNING OBJECTS

LINA PETRAKIEVA ■ DICKSON NEILSON TELFER ■
DAVID McARTHUR

## CHAPTER OUTLINE

## OBJECTIVES

*This chapter should support the reader to develop an understanding of:*

- Planning, designing, and creating reusable learning objects (RLOs)
- Selecting software packages and web platforms to suit your needs
- Ways to enhance learner engagement when using the RLO
- Ways to overcome common pitfalls when producing media sources for your RLO
- Ways RLOs can be used to support simulation-based education

## KEY TERMS

| | |
|---|---|
| **Reusable learning objects (RLOs)** | **Blended learning** |
| **Learning objects** | **Technology enhanced learning** |

## INTRODUCTION

As more and more content is being delivered online, the reusable learning object (RLO) has become an increasingly popular feature in contemporary higher education. In a time where it is no longer uncommon for institutions to offer several courses part-time and/or via distance learning, topped up by the significant increase in online delivery during the

COVID-19 outbreak of 2020 and 2021, the popularity and educational importance of the RLO comes as no surprise. However, not unlike email, unless the content is well-planned, carefully considered and executed, with the target audience in mind, misinterpretation or misunderstanding can occur. Add to this the potential hazards and time associated with navigating unfamiliar software or platforms, and it can become an all-encompassing task that falls into the 'it seemed like a good idea at the time' category. This chapter will assist you in carrying out the required thinking and planning to ensure your RLO is accessible and useful to your target audience and beyond. Between them, the authors have many years of experience creating RLOs and ensuring they are engaging, informative and, above all, reusable. The advice will be imparted in mainly generic terms but will also touch upon RLOs for simulation-based education (SBE).

## BACKGROUND

RLOs can be defined and described in many ways, but in essence they are digital, structured learning objects with a focus on a single learning objective using multimedia and sound pedagogical principles. Many use Gagne and Medsker's (1996) nine key instructional events: gaining learners' attention, highlighting key features, structured learning, presenting content, learner guidance, eliciting performance, providing feedback, assessing performance, and enhancing retention and transfer; however, this is by no means a rule.

Although any digital learning material such as videos, pdf files, and so on could be considered as learning objects, it is important to acknowledge that these resources are static containers of information, not easily reusable, and definitely not interactive for effective user engagement. Effective learning objects should provide elements of information utilising various formats (text, audio, video, etc.), should engage users with interactive content and opportunities for self-assessment, and should provide feedback. Therefore, an effective RLO will need to be constructed in such a way that its design incorporates the elements discussed earlier, while ensuring the content and delivery structure are easy to modify and repurpose.

## CONTEXT

When designing and creating an RLO, it is important to consider how regularly it will be reused. There is little point in spending 12 hours to create something that will benefit a cohort of 15 students for a single module, especially if it is a module that is subject to regular or semi-regular change. For example, if your target audience consists of learners in health and life sciences disciplines, it is recommended that you consider the likelihood of changes in content in line with government or professional body requirements. This may lead you to design an RLO with the knowledge that an update will be necessary at some point, or it may inform a more generic, universal approach to your design. Regardless, the end user must be the primary consideration; if your RLO has a shelf-life, it may be worthwhile indicating this at some point, even if it is in the small print. You do not want to find yourself in a position where you have to redesign regularly (the R, after all, stands for reusable), but at the same time it may be unrealistic to expect any learning resource to have infinite relevance. The subject discipline, the focus, and the design of the RLO will likely dictate its expected shelf-life.

Ideally, you want to create something once that will be used on many occasions, for a reasonable period of time, and by a large number of learners. If it does not contain relevant and pertinent module content, or refers to potentially outdated practices, theories, and references, you will find yourself spending unnecessary time revisiting it to address these avoidable mistakes. Planning and design are therefore imperative to the usability and success of your RLO.

To maximise the effectiveness, the timing of the deployment is crucial as learners are more likely to engage if it is tailored and time relevant for the point of need for the subject or topic being studied. The RLO can be made available permanently (always on) or it can be 'released' at the point of need. If it is always on, it could be useful for those whose study pattern differs from the main course cohort or when the course design is flexible and includes participants from different time zones; however, it may also become viewed as a 'background' and be ignored. If 'released' in a timed relevant manner to coincide with the course curriculum requirement, then learner 'buy-in' may improve engagement and learning. Potentially, it can also be made available but highlighted at a relevant point in the study process to get the benefit of both.

The content itself ideally should be designed to be seen as contextualised or tailored so that learners can better relate to it and readily apply the knowledge. However, this approach could reduce the shelf-life and reusability of the RLO. Making the content generic though, would require the learners to evaluate and apply the generic knowledge learned to their circumstances and studies, so they may be disenfranchised from the whole experience of engaging with the RLO (Fig. 2.1).

This is not to say that you should not design an RLO for a small cohort of students, but if they are on campus every week and you have regular contact with them, it might be best to deliver the content face-to-face rather than through an RLO. Of course, an RLO could be used to supplement your teaching, by way of short information and a quiz or drag and drop activity to reinforce learning, and to allow the learners to formatively self-assess.

In summary, before you decide to build an RLO, carefully consider the following:

- Learner numbers (large enough cohort)
- The universality of your RLO (reusability of the RLO)

- Timelessness (if appropriate) – make the resource as long-term as possible
- Learner needs (do learners need this RLO)

## PLANNING A REUSABLE LEARNING OBJECT

Frustration and exasperation are often the result when teaching staff see evidence of learners not paying due attention to an assignment brief. Sometimes it can appear to assessment markers that learners have read the assignment brief only once and then jumped straight in without doing sufficient reading, research, planning, and drafting. Similarly, it is important that the designer of an RLO adopts the same approach they expect (or hope) their learners will take. Planning around content, intention, academic level, and software or platform choice are all important considerations before putting something together (Fig. 2.2).

When considering how to develop an RLO and what platform to use, there are several considerations that should be taken into account:

1. Who are the target audience, and what are their needs?
2. Who will be using it, and what study year/level will the RLO be pitched at?
3. Where will they be using it?

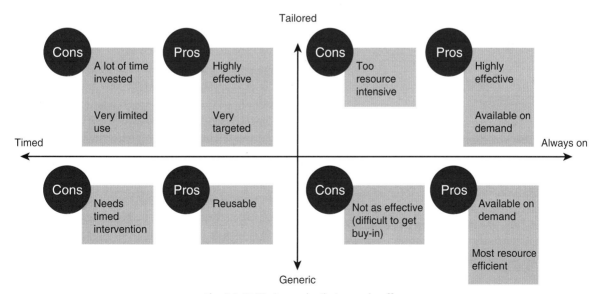

**Fig. 2.1** ■ Timing and tailoring trade-offs.

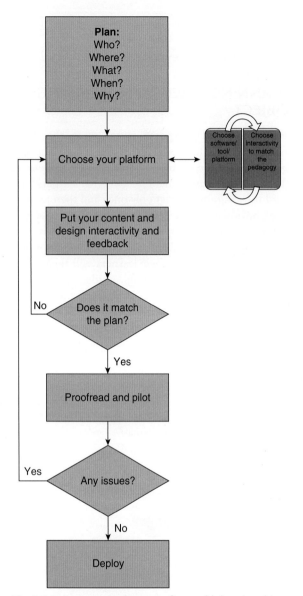

**Fig. 2.2** ■ Stages in development of a reusable learning object.

4. Will internet access be required for online use?
5. Will downloading be required for offline use?
6. What content will be conveyed?
7. When and how often do they need to access it, i.e., is it for study, revision, or for reference?
8. What is the purpose and goal of the RLO (topic)?

It is a good idea to write down your answers to these eight questions. These can be utilised as iterative

guidelines after you have created your draft RLO, to check if it matches your plan and adjust accordingly.

## CHOOSING A PLATFORM/ SOFTWARE FOR THE DEVELOPMENT OF A REUSABLE LEARNING OBJECT

Just when you thought the groundwork and preparatory element of your RLO planning was complete, another particularly important element rears its head. What tool/software/platform will best suit the creation of your interactive RLO resource, and how and where will your RLO be accessed. This section offers what could be the more confusing element of RLO development, including encouraging consideration of which software package or web platform will offer the best solution for the creation of your interactive and informative RLO content.

### Internet Access

Your internet access could be a factor in determining whether you use a design software (physically downloaded and available from your computer) or a web-based platform, accessible through an internet browser.

### Institutional Support

Does the institution support the software or design platform you want to use? Is there already an existing licence and/or technical support for the platform or software you are planning to use?

### Licence

There are multiple types of licences, and the potential cost implications could be the single most key factor to consider when deciding which platform or software to use. There are free platforms and tools, but they usually add adverts to help the creators pay the cost of creation and maintenance, and those adverts may make the final RLO look unprofessional. They may also be free because they are new and/or a pilot and, as such, they may not be bug-free or established enough to stay live for a reasonable period of time. The last thing anyone needs is to spend a long time building something using software or a platform that disappears in a few months. It could also be possible to buy a perpetual licence which provides access to the software or platform for as long as it is supported by the creator. This allows for planning costs and potential savings, but it may end up creating an RLO using technology that could become out of date or incompatible due to the ever changing and evolving digital world. Another option could be the purchase of a subscription licence, which means that there will be a regular payment of money every month or year. This type of licence also provides continual updates which ensures access to the newest technologies on offer from that creator.

### Interactivity Offered/Needed

When planning an RLO the pedagogy should be the driver for selecting the type of interactivity to be added to the design; however, each software/platform will offer a separate set of interactive options which may or may not include the types that you had considered for your design. They may also offer interactive options that you have not considered, and which could inspire you and provide an opportunity to rethink the design and types of interactivities to be used within the RLO.

If the RLO is intended to be used multiple times with the same audience, for example for revision purposes, then a more sophisticated interactive design may be required (i.e., one that allows for randomisation).

### Longevity

In the digital world, everything changes eventually and/or disappears; however, when choosing a software or platform for creating an RLO, there are basic checks that could be carried out to help optimise the chances of it being available and suitable for the longest period possible. Careful research of the provider's history will offer some insight on whether the company is small and/or new to the market or is bigger and longer established. The platform/software history also needs to be considered as some projects from bigger established companies may not last, whereas some of the newer companies to the market may offer more up-to-date technologies and fresh ideas. There are never any guarantees for the possible futures of any provider/creator or the platform/software they offer. However, it is always prudent to exercise common sense and to ensure that backups are kept, as will be discussed later in this chapter.

### Access

Once the RLO has been created, it is important to consider how it will be accessed by learners, that is, is it intended for download for use offline or will it be accessed from online using an internet browser? It is vital to ensure that the software/platform allows for the appropriate access method. If the RLO is intended to be downloaded, then it can simply be placed in the virtual learning environment (VLE) or a network repository where learners can download as required. However, if the RLO will be web accessible, as most educational resources of this nature tend to be, the hosting requirements of the RLO need to be considered. Hosting refers to the online or web-based server storage that provides access to the RLO content. Most web-based design platforms will usually provide a hosting service automatically; however, this is not a guaranteed provision and needs to be properly checked. Some institutions may provide internal hosting servers, which may be another option to explore. However, learner access from off campus locations should also be checked because some institutional hosting servers may only provide on campus access.

Once all of this is determined, it is then a case of finding the most suitable software or platform for the creation of the RLO. Multiple lists of current software/platforms can be found online together with feedback from users and that offer a good starting point for the selection of a software/platform that will best suit your requirements. No list or recommendations of specific software/platforms are included within this chapter as accessing a list of potential resources at the point of need will ensure you are able to use the most up-to-date resources.

## CONTENT DESIGN

An RLO should provide an introduction, a brief outline of the content, and/or a (short) list of learning outcome(s) which should clearly indicate the intention of the RLO and what the learner should expect to have knowledge of once they have worked through it. Learning outcome(s) should be clear and concise, making effective use of instructive words and phrases such as 'determine', 'prioritise', 'apply the principles of', and so on. Depending on how much detail you want to provide, you could also map the learning outcomes to the relevant graduate attributes criteria.

Usually, an RLO will only cover a limited volume of content so the introduction and/or learning outcomes can look like surplus material. Therefore it is your judgement call as to whether it is appropriate, and where this detail should be incorporated. Be conscious though that (in theory) RLOs should be lively, colourful (where appropriate), engaging, and interactive; they are not merely glorified PowerPoints with the occasional voiceover and photograph. Like any piece of academic work, an RLO should have an obvious beginning, middle, and end.

It is also particularly important to consider that an RLO needs to be self-sufficient, offering the learner all relevant materials without the need for additional help or information from academic staff. Ideally the RLO should be self-contained as much as possible to maintain learner focus and to avoid directing them to external resources that are not within your editorial control and/or likely to change or be removed. However, where possible, learners should be directed to external sources if they are likely to always contain the most up-to-date information rather than having to personally edit the RLO with every change. For example, if you want to show your learners how they should engage with social media as a health professional, it would be better to include a link directly to the relevant professional body's document for that, rather than replicating the content within the RLO.

In terms of the academic study level for whom the RLO is intended, it may be appropriate to indicate this in or near the opening section of your RLO. In some cases, this may not be necessary, for example if the RLO is being uploaded onto a private VLE for a particular cohort of students. However, if you are exporting it to a central server and making the link available to the wider world, or uploading it to a website where anyone can access the RLO, it may be worthwhile informing users of the intended target audience.

## INTERACTIVITY

As previously discussed, a good RLO should include interactivity and/or self-assessment with feedback. Depending on the content to be included, you may wish to incorporate self-assessment elements throughout your RLO, or you may opt to include one at the end.

These could be in the form of quiz questions with feedback, that is, the learner should not only be informed if they are correct or not (they could have guessed!), they should also be informed as to why they are correct (supplying supportive confirmation of their knowledge), or why they are incorrect (so that learners can address their area(s) for development). As part of this, it may be useful to add links to other resources that provide thorough explanations and more examples and so on. It is also important to ensure that any links open in separate pages or tabs; it can be very frustrating for the user to have to reload the RLO and then find their way back to the section they were engaging with.

Any RLOs in which the user selects the incorrect answer and are simply told they are wrong, then asked to answer the question again, equates to nothing more than the online equivalent of a verbal rebuke. Therefore, this type of approach to interactive design and content will not necessarily lead to a good learning outcome. As an example, an RLO was created by one of the chapter authors on the topic of referencing using an open-source application called Xerte. This RLO is quiz-based but includes a variety of question types, for example, true or false; pick all that apply; how many of the following . . . and so on. One of the questions asked, 'Can I use Twitter as a reference?' The answer options are simply 'Yes' or 'No' but selecting either answer generates new content. If 'Yes' is selected, the user is told they are correct, informed why they are correct, and then provided with a short video which shows the parameters, rules, and format of referencing a tweet. Similarly, if the user selects 'No', they are informed they are incorrect, given reasons, and again directed to a short video (Fig. 2.3).

This is a good example, because although it is a yes or no question, there are a few things which reinforce or clarify the learning, in particular the video. The video talks about quality control, that is, referencing a tweet from a random member of the public who has a strong opinion on something is not considered academic, and therefore not suitable for academic purposes. However, a tweet from a recognised academic or researcher, or indeed a conversation between a student and a professor of nursing studies, who does regular TED talks on the topic, is deemed appropriate, and therefore suitable for referencing in an academic piece of work. Having

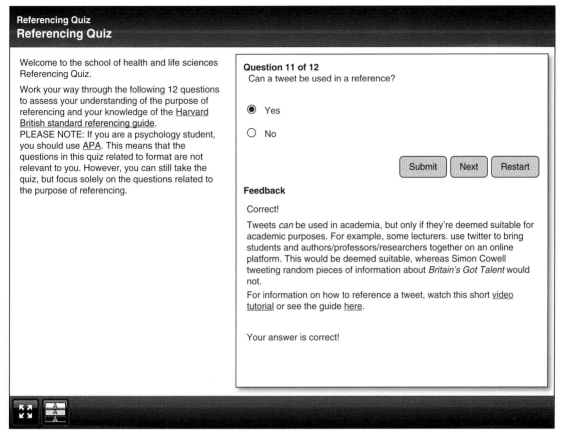

**Referencing Quiz**
**Referencing Quiz**

Welcome to the school of health and life sciences Referencing Quiz.

Work your way through the following 12 questions to assess your understanding of the purpose of referencing and your knowledge of the Harvard British standard referencing guide.
PLEASE NOTE: If you are a psychology student, you should use APA. This means that the questions in this quiz related to format are not relevant to you. However, you can still take the quiz, but focus solely on the questions related to the purpose of referencing.

**Question 11 of 12**
Can a tweet be used in a reference?

◉ Yes

○ No

Submit   Next   Restart

**Feedback**

Correct!

Tweets *can* be used in academia, but only if they're deemed suitable for academic purposes. For example, some lecturers. use twitter to bring students and authors/professors/researchers together on an online platform. This would be deemed suitable, whereas Simon Cowell tweeting random pieces of information about *Britain's Got Talent* would not.

For information on how to reference a tweet, watch this short video tutorial or see the guide here.

Your answer is correct!

**Fig. 2.3** ■ Referencing quiz RLO designed using Xerte. *RLO,* Reusable learning object.

been led through this process, the learner has experienced interactivity, self-assessment, feedback, and further guidance through a short, friendly, audio-visual explanation (incorporating colour, tone, inflection, and emphasis). This ensures that those who are correct know why that is the case, those who are incorrect learn where they went wrong, and those who adopted the potluck 50/50 approach are also swept into the mix. This process therefore considers pedagogical principles whilst delivering the content in ways that are arguably more engaging and impactful than merely reading the referencing guide or a white A4 handout with black text that says yes, tweets can be referenced but there are rules.

To ensure your RLO is active (and interactive) rather than passive, it is recommended to include images or diagrams and/or videos or sound clips. Again, this seems obvious, and there is no need to have all of these

on each page/slide, but flipping between text, diagrams, audio, video, and interactivity will maximise your chances of user engagement and, as a result – in theory at least – knowledge, understanding, and application (Ibrahim and Al-Shara, 2007). Essentially, make it as appealing and playful as possible, incorporating an appropriate level of gamification to engage learners whilst adhering to pedagogical principles, relevance, and academic level.

## DURATION AND ATTENTION SPAN

When planning and developing an RLO it is important to carefully consider the length of time users will be expected to engage with the resource. Even the most interesting of subject matter requires concentration to absorb information from, which can in itself cause fatigue. There are various theories regarding the average person's concentration/attention span, with Elsworthy (2017) reporting that it is between 14 and 29 minutes. However, due to the ever-increasing number of distractions in the modern world, this may be lower for some learners, as low as seven minutes (Agarwal, 2021). For learners with disabilities such as dyslexia, Meares-Irlen syndrome, and attention deficit hyperactive disorder, it may also be the case that ability to concentrate is compromised after only a few minutes. This does, however, depend on the degree of investment the learner has with the topic and - very importantly – how dynamic and engaging the delivery is (Bradbury, 2016).

An effective way to maintain user concentration and engagement with the RLO is to interject interactive tasks, where users can become physically and mentally engaged with content while, at the same time, change from the passive mode of information absorption. Active engagement within an RLO is a primary feature of online learning and can improve learner satisfaction with their learning process.

While designing the RLO, the duration of interaction should be considered simultaneously with the complexity of the information being presented. The more complex the subject matter is, the deeper the concentration that is required, therefore reducing the time it can be maintained. Concentration times can be improved with careful structuring of complex content, arranging the detail into more easily absorbed 'chunks', and with the injection of interactive tasks where natural breaks of information delivery are present.

## MEDIA PRODUCTION ADVICE AND ACCESSIBILITY

Firstly, if the blended learning, marketing, and/or audio-visual departments in your school/faculty/institution offer filming, audio recording, or photographic services to staff, it makes sense to contact them – they will have more experience and better equipment, which will help get the job done more quickly and will make your RLO look more professional.

Should you need to undertake the creation of your own media, then following the hints, tips, and guidelines below should help you in the creation of effective and professional standard materials.

### Importance of Acquiring Participant Consent

If recording or involving other people for your resources (video, audio, images, or text) you should obtain their written consent to use the recordings or materials generated, and clearly state how the materials will be used. Consider the following example:

A course leader wanted to develop a resource to help learners prepare for a final examination in the format of an Objective Structured Clinical Exam (OSCE). In an attempt to make this authentic for the learner, the course leader had the idea to design a learning object that included video footage of a real example of a poor OSCE performance. They planned to produce a resource which was captioned and included quiz questions which would tie in with the assessment rubric.

While this may sound like a great way of tangibly demonstrating to students where things can go wrong in their upcoming OSCE, we would need to consider if it would be appropriate or indeed ethical to approach a student who had failed an examination and ask to use their footage for this purpose. Even if the student had given verbal consent initially, without written consent this footage could not be used. Would it be any wonder if consent was refused by a student who may have concerns about sharing their poor performance with hundreds, perhaps thousands of other/future students?

Although the intentions of the course leader were good, there was a lack of consideration of how potentially damaging it could be for the student in question. Furthermore, we must ask ourselves if showing poor practice and performance is a positive learning tool, as it runs the risk of confusing learners.

When using footage, it may be a safer option to use actors such as members of staff willing to help recreate a learning situation. This should be carefully planned and rehearsed though, with clear guidance provided to all involved and written consent obtained where required.

### Video

There are a few things to consider if including video in your RLO for technical skills. Video materials for learning and teaching do not have to be cinema standard; however, it is important to avoid recording fuzzy, out-of-focus images or creating a two-shot conversation, where two people are in the one frame, and cutting out part of one participant's face. Here are some fundamental guidelines you could consider following to achieve a better-quality video:

**Light** – Ensure that light (sunlight in particular) is coming from behind the camera, or if portable lighting sources are used, diffusers are utilised to even out the light intensity and reduce shadows.

**Framing** – Ensure that video is recorded in landscape orientation, and ideally in widescreen (16:9) format. The main object being filmed should be the largest and dominant subject of the frame. If filming people and faces, make sure that you only leave a little bit of space above their head. You can find more tips on framing online as the guidelines will depend on the object being filmed and the purpose of the video.

**Resolution** – Record in the highest resolution available on the camera, which will allow you to reframe during editing without losing a lot of the resolution. Ideally you would want the final video to be in full high definition (HD) (1920 × 1080). You may, however, have to consider file size implications if the video is to be viewed by learners who do not have good internet access, or speed, to either download or stream it.

**Sound** – When recording video, be mindful of the audio quality. It is always best to use a good quality microphone with a wind screen or muff, particularly when recording outdoors. It is also important to listen for background sound (for example wind or fans) or noises (whining hard drive noise, computer fans, etc.) which could affect and/or cause distraction during playback. Using background music or sound effects during the editing process can help conceal unwanted audio anomalies; however, avoiding recording those is always the better option.

**Focus** – Always ensure the camera has been properly focussed on the primary subject. Blurred video recordings do not hold viewer attention. Keep images sharp, and where possible, ensure that people being filmed remain stationary to make sure camera focus does not drift.

**Angle** – Ideally you want to film directly opposite the object, rather than from a very high or very low perspective, as it will feel more natural and more like the viewer is seeing it with their own eyes.

**Dress code** – Although it may seem superficial, consider what you (and anyone else in the footage) should wear. How do you want to be perceived by your learners? Will you potentially be showcasing this RLO at a conference? If yes, how do you want to be perceived by your peers, both internal and external? Try not to shoot footage the day before a badly needed haircut or the day after an experimental haircut that has turned out not quite how you expected or are pleased with. Remember, your RLO, once complete and uploaded, may become the property of the institution you work for and could therefore be on the internet for the rest of (your) time.

Remember, accessibility laws in the United Kingdom require that you should always provide accompanying captions (subtitles) or a downloadable transcript.

## Audio

It is more difficult to maintain concentration when listening on audio only, so if using audio clips, make them short and to the point. When recording audio for narration, interviews, or any other scenario, the same basic advice applies as with video: use a good quality microphone with a wind screen or muff; and listen for background sound or noises which could affect and/or cause distraction during playback.

Microphone technique is also very important. If a microphone is held too close to the subject, there is a strong possibility of recording breathing noises and/or pop and scratch anomalies from lips and skin contact. If the microphone is held too far away from the subject, the audio recording quality will be reduced and potentially produce audio that is unusable. As a rough guideline, microphones should be kept at a distance of 10 to 15 cm from the subject. However, it is always good practice to test record samples before making a final production recording.

Once again, please remember, accessibility law requires that you should always provide accompanying captions (subtitles) or a downloadable transcript.

## Images/Graphics

Ideally you should own any images you use within the RLO. Any photographic images required should be taken by you with a good-quality camera to ensure that they are not copyrighted and will be exactly as you want them. However, if you need to find your images from other sources, you need to make sure that the image is legal to be used (check licences) and that it is of sufficient quality and good resolution to be able to display the level of detail you require. Any diagrams or charts will need to be created using an appropriate software application (PowerPoint, Visio, Excel, etc.) to achieve good quality and to match your needs. It is always a good idea to keep the original or master file and format of the diagram or chart, and to save edited versions when any changes need to be made. Then save or export a picture version (jpg, gif, etc.) of the diagram/chart being used in the RLO.

In keeping with accessibility laws, always ensure that all images used have additional 'alt-text' attribute information attached to accurately describe the image content or purpose (action button). This is particularly important for chart representation images or diagrams. Tables of information ideally should be recreated for delivering that information in the RLO rather than being presented in an image format. Attempting to describe a table within an alt-text attribute would not be an effective or time efficient way to make the information accessible.

## Text

Although the RLO is usually designed for the purposes of delivering complex information, usually based on a single topic, the included text needs to be kept succinct. Text should be interlaced with supporting imagery and/or multimedia resources to further enhance the information delivery and knowledge acquisition. It is important to avoid unnecessary abbreviations and acronyms while keeping the phraseology simple and easy to understand, without losing the important academic nature of the topic. This will assist learners to comfortably and successfully engage with the content.

## Fonts, Colours, and Overall Design

An RLO is digital in nature so this will have an influence when choosing which fonts will be used. As sans-serif fonts, including Calibri, Arial, Verdana, Tahoma, and so on, offer a clearer reading experience on screen they should always be the first choice for screen presentation, rather than a serif font like Times New Roman. As a guideline you should never use more than two different fonts in one piece of work, that is, one for heading and one for the main text.

Consider the devices and circumstances in which the learners will engage with the RLO and make sure that your minimum font size is appropriate. It is always a good idea to test how the RLO will look on different devices to ensure it is fit for purpose.

When designing an RLO, the choice of colour(s) is a complex problem to address. There are lots of different aspects to consider and sometimes they may be contradictory. For example, ideally you would like to achieve best contrast, but should avoid using just black and white (which is the best contrast you could achieve). The use of corporate colours (or colour schemes) may be a good route to consider; however, also think about the appropriateness of those colours in terms of content and cultural significance for your learners. As an example, if the corporate colour option available is bright pink, but your RLO is about grief counselling, it may not be the best idea to use such a cheerful colour for it.

As a basic guideline, use a light background with a dark font and colours that will look appealing and appropriate. If you choose to utilise colours to colour-code information, make sure that you consider any potential accessibility issues (like colour deficiency); ensure that the information coding is supplemented by additional notation, that is, if group A is coded with blue and group B is coded with green, make sure that you also include the identifiers 'A' and 'B' and not just the colours to distinguish between the two.

As an example, a series of RLOs was requested for students from Singapore, with one of the requirements being that the design should be colourful. When a rationale was requested for this, the advice provided was that the general learning preferences of the culture was that of colourful resources, and that the these would be instrumental in terms of maximising concentration. On reflection, this made sense, given the choice between interacting with something colourful and engaging or black text on white paper/background, one would be more likely to choose the colourful option. This changed our perspective and made us realise there is no reason 'complex' academic topics cannot be presented using a spectrum of vibrant colours to enhance engagement and recall (Dzulkifli and Mustafar, 2013).

## Improving Reusability

An increase of an RLO shelf-life can easily be achieved with careful planning. Here are a few things to consider:

- If possible, avoid referring to resources or codes of practice that are updated on a regular basis with their dates or editions, for example. when mentioning APA referencing style, use 'APA referencing style' rather than 'APA referencing style version 7'.
- Do not mention specific details, for example, rooms, buildings, phone numbers, email addresses, points of contact, individual members of staff. All of these are subject to change, so try to keep things generic where possible. If contact details are required for the RLO, use a generic email address that can be accessed by multiple team members.
- If the RLO is hosted on a network or web-based platform and uses an email address for user registration or contact, use a generic email address. This also ensures that any change of staffing responsible for updating and maintaining the RLO content still have access.
- Any information that is time sensitive and cannot be avoided using the previously mentioned methods should be kept to one specific place/ section in the RLO. This ensures that any editing of this information is kept to a minimum within the RLO and prevents missing any instances that could potentially be embedded throughout.
- Unless necessary, avoid referring to specific pieces of software, for example, say 'VLE' or 'virtual learning environment' rather than 'Moodle' or 'Blackboard'. This will date your RLO.
- If you use video in your RLO which features real people (this may include you), take into consideration that the footage may be watched on several occasions by large audiences. If you intend to make the RLO an Open Educational Resource (OER) or release it under a Creative Commons licence, and put it online for widespread use, avoid using dated expressions, or exhibiting fake behaviour that has no place in clinical practice.
- Ensure backup files for all elements of media that are used within the RLO are kept in one or more separate storage spaces. This safeguards any loss of RLO access through platform issues or user access issue (loss of access rights, passwords, etc.).

## REUSABLE LEARNING OBJECTS IN SIMULATION-BASED EDUCATION

RLOs in simulation-based education (SBE) lend themselves to a combination of video and interactivity. Envisage a split screen; in the left panel there could be some textual information and a video clip of, for example, a nursing student engaging with a patient (played by an actor, staff member, or fellow student) or a Manikin/ patient simulator with the text providing some basic information and instructions; the right panel contains a quiz question or an activity. Following the guidelines mentioned earlier in this chapter, ensure that feedback provided for the question or activity covers both correct and incorrect responses. Alternatively, there may be a 'drag and drop' activity or 'fill in the blanks' activity. Add some colour and vibrancy to the page, and you are already tapping into a considerable proportion of what constitutes a successful RLO (Fig. 2.4).

When assessing breathing, the nurse reports the child has stridor. What is 'stridor'?

a. A high-pitched noise usually on expiration

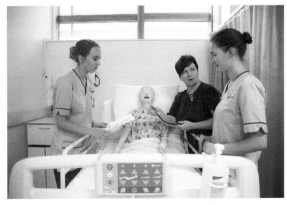

**Fig. 2.4** ■ Manikin/patient simulator.

b. A whistling sound usually on inspiration

c. A high-pitched noise usually on inspiration

d. A coarse rattling respiratory sound

e. A whistling sound usually on expiration

f. A rattling sound on inspiration

Within SBE, there are plenty of opportunities to include this kind of content to help ensure the correct messages are communicated to the target audience in a non-passive, non-didactic fashion.

## TOP TIPS

| Top Tip | Guidance |
|---|---|
| ■ **Make the reusable learning object (RLO) 'reusable'** | Remember planning and design are vital to the usability and success of your RLO. Depending on the subject, you may be designing an RLO with the knowledge that an update will be necessary at some point. However, a more generic, universal approach to your design may improve longevity. As the end user must be the primary consideration, if your RLO has a shelf-life (e.g., resuscitation guidelines), it is worth acknowledging this at some point, even if it is in the small print.<br><br>Strategies such as including URL links to sites with documents or guidelines, rather than the document itself, can mean when these are updated, the learner may be directed to the latest version. |
| ■ **Improving learner engagement with material** | Learners are more likely to engage if the RLO is tailored and time relevant for the point of need for the subject or topic being studied. Options are either making the RLO available permanently (always on) or it can be 'released' at the point of need. While RLOs which are 'always on' could be useful for those who require flexible study, there is a risk it may become a 'background' and easily ignored. Releasing the RLO to coincide with the course curriculum requirement, may improve engagement and learning. |
| ■ **Selecting the best platform to host your RLO** | Do your homework! Research the software/platform provider's background to find out if the company is small and/or new to the market or if it is a more established, larger operation. Look at the provider's history as some projects from bigger established companies may not last, whereas newer companies may offer more up-to-date technologies and fresh ideas. There are never any guarantees for the possible futures of any provider or the software they provide; therefore, it is always wise to ensure that backups are kept. |

| Top Tip | Guidance |
|---|---|
| ■ **RLO on the go: facilitating learner access** | You need to decide if this is to be downloaded or web accessible. Web accessible can offer more flexibility but you need to check whether the web-based design platform provides a hosting service. |
| ■ **Making it interactive and safe to make mistakes** | Activities such as self-assessment either throughout or at the end of your RLO can keep the learner actively involved and engaged. If you decide to use quiz questions with feedback, remember learners may guess the answer. Therefore, in addition to letting them know if they are correct or not, you should also provide information to why they are correct (supplying supportive confirmation of their knowledge), or why they are incorrect (so that learners can address their area(s) for development). |

## SUMMARY

Although RLOs have been in use for academic purposes for some considerable time, the impact of the COVID-19 pandemic has resulted in a significant impact and uptake in online digital learning and teaching. Consequently, there has been an increased awareness and interest in the use of RLOs within programmes of study that had not previously considered such technologies for distance learning and teaching opportunities. Once a digital approach has been adopted, the return to only face-to-face learning and teaching methods becomes almost unthinkable.

As such, it is anticipated that a more blended approach will be the way forward within health and social care, and academic institutions, with online teaching and support continuing alongside on-campus input, tutorials, practical activities, and assessments. This will mean an increased need for more high-quality RLO development, as this will allow for asynchronous delivery of content that learners can access in a more flexible way. From the perspective of SBE, this therefore places increased importance on RLOs to be of high quality, that is, engaging, attractive, clear, useful, interactive, and informative to the hundreds or even thousands of learners who will access and benefit from them.

Although some elements of health and social care practice can never be fully replicated through a digital approach, the forced rapid switch to online learning during the pandemic also meant that many of the teaching approaches or activities, previously considered to be only possible in a face-to-face environment (e.g., clinical skills), have now become more flexible in their approach. This will hopefully encourage practitioners to reconsider how they approach their teaching practices in terms of the use of SBE.

## REFERENCES

Agarwal, N., 2021. Can you focus beyond 7 minutes? [WWW Document]. Team Toppr. Available at: https://teamtoppr.medium.com/can-you-focus-beyond-7-minutes-bcc6f3b7c202. (Accessed 22 July 2021).

Bradbury, N.A., 2016. Attention span during lectures: 8 seconds, 10 minutes, or more? Adv. Physiol. Educ. 40, 509–513.

Dzulkifli, M.A., Mustafar, M.F., 2013. The influence of colour on memory performance: a review. Malays. J. Med. Sci. 20, 3–9.

Elsworthy, E., 2017. Average British attention span is 14 minutes, research finds | The Independent | The Independent [WWW Document]. Independent. Available at: https://www.independent.co.uk/news/uk/home-news/attention-span-average-british-person-tuned-concentration-mobile-phone-a8131156.html. (Accessed 22 July 2021).

Gagne and Medsker, 1996. The conditions of learning: training applications. Harcourt and Bruce: San Diego, California.

Ibrahim, M., Al-Shara, O., 2007. Impact of interactive learning on knowledge retention. Lect. Notes Comput. Sci. (including Subser. Lect. Notes Artif. Intell. Lect. Notes Bioinformatics) 4558 LNCS, 347–355.

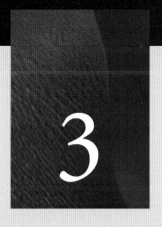

# 3

# DEVELOPING A FACULTY FOR EFFECTIVE IMMERSIVE SIMULATION

CATIE PATON ▪ ELIZABETH SIMPSON ▪ GAYLE ANN MACKIE ▪ DANIEL LYNAGH ▪ ZOE HUTCHESON

## CHAPTER OUTLINE

## OBJECTIVES

*This chapter should support the reader to develop an understanding of the:*

- Roles and responsibilities of the individual faculty team members
- Educational theories which apply to simulation-based education (SBE)
- Development process involved in becoming a simulation faculty member
- Planning, delivery, and evaluation of a faculty development programme
- Stages of a simulation session and skills required for effective simulation briefing, scenario delivery, and simulation debriefing
- Continuing professional development of faculty and the role this plays in sustaining faculty

## KEY TERMS

Coach

Co-facilitation

Co-ordintator

Debrief

Debriefer

Embedded professional

Facilitation

Facilitator

Faculty development

Feedback

Immersive simulation

Meta debrief

Novice faculty

Simulated patient

Simulation educator

Simulation faculty development

Simulation technician

## INTRODUCTION

Simulation is a practical way to learn, develop, and generally enhance skills for a wide range of health and care professionals. This educational approach is grounded in learning theories (Aebersold, 2018), with the principal aim of enhancing the delivery of safe and effective person-centred care.

Currently, health and care professions adopt simulation as a strategy for learning, across a range of activities from acquisition of practical skills to immersive simulation scenarios. This approach allows learners to practice in a safe environment and reflect on their experience, avoiding unnecessary risk to patients. The most effective way to generate a safe, positive learning environment which harnesses the ethos of simulation-based education (SBE) is to develop a faculty of experts. These experts should have an appreciation of the educational theories which underpin SBE, including constructivism, experiential learning, and reflection.

This chapter will share practical advice on how to develop and establish a faculty to deliver simulation and will also explore the importance of collaboration within the faculty team. The chapter will also include a case study which focuses on a one-day development course for novice simulation faculty. This one-day course is part of a faculty development programme which includes ongoing Continuing Professional Development (CPD) activities to facilitate maintenance of the faculty's skills.

## BACKGROUND

Historically, simulation faculty development has been challenging as a consequence of the evolving nature of the health and care environment. However, it is a worthwhile exercise, despite the challenges, as developing an expert simulation faculty who can respond to the ever-changing requirements of contemporary health and care systems can positively influence both the quality of the simulation delivered and the subsequent care which is provided (Lateef, 2010). As the demand for SBE grows as a strategy to develop health and care professionals, establishing an expert simulation faculty is increasingly recognised as a priority, effectively helping to ensure that core teams can be established to support the delivery of these simulation programmes.

Faculty teamwork and collaboration are pivotal to the successful delivery of SBE. The roles within the simulation faculty will therefore most likely be varied and could include educators, technologists, embedded professionals, and administrators. However, depending on your area, and the staff and resources available, some team members may be required to undertake several roles concurrently. Irrespective of this, and to ensure parity in the learner experience, a standardised approach to faculty development is required. This chapter will therefore be reflective of our own experiences of developing a sustainable simulation faculty and will provide an overview of the continuing professional development process aligned with each role.

## CONTEXT

Health and care disciplines already recognise the effectiveness of simulation as a teaching and learning strategy. Because of this, the need for consistency, quality assurance, and appropriately structured and standardised preparation are recognised as essential when preparing staff to support the delivery of SBE programmes (Decker et al., 2015; Eppich and Cheng, 2015; Jeffries et al., 2015). Developing and sustaining a team of expert simulation faculty members will require investment in the team and the provision of ongoing CPD programmes. A number of UK, European, and international simulation education organisations have produced standards for delivery of SBE programmes and, in particular, highlight the role of faculty development in the maintenance of simulation activity quality assurance (Decker et al., 2013, 2015; Franklin et al., 2013; Sitiner et al., 2015).

Ideally, the structure of simulation faculty development courses should mirror the structure of the actual simulation learning process. Unsurprisingly, parallels can therefore be drawn between preparing to become a simulation faculty member and the mastery learning process. Outlined in more detail as part of Chapters 4 and 5, mastery learning acknowledges the individuality of learners, recognising that the speed at which they develop skills will differ. Alongside this, it is also recognised that practise in isolation does not produce experts. To achieve mastery requires a period of deliberate practice with timeous, constructive feedback to inform the individual's reflection. Following this approach when preparing faculty should take the prospective faculty member on the journey from novice to expert.

## Faculty Roles and Responsibilities

The roles and responsibilities of faculty members will be determined by their stage on the development journey. Table 3.1 provides an overview of faculty members' roles, their responsibilities, and their contributions, within a simulation team. The associated characteristics, attributes, behaviours, and skills are also presented, while taking into consideration the level of experience required for each role.

### Time Out: Your Team

Take time to think about your team, and the roles and responsibilities they could adopt. (Tip: think about their existing talents and try to align roles and responsibilities with these strengths.)

It is now clear that the roles and responsibilities of each member of the simulation faculty are both wide ranging and, at times, overlapping. As a faculty delivering simulation, it is therefore important to have some appreciation of how adults learn. This will help to ensure that the discharge of each of the roles, and the learning and teaching strategies more generally, are focused on promoting learner engagement.

## TEACHING, LEARNING, AND ASSESSMENT STRATEGIES

Biggs and Tang (2011) present three levels of thinking aligned with teaching, presenting the notion that the effectiveness of teaching is related to our interpretation and understanding of what we believe teaching is (Table 3.2). The first two levels of thinking are rooted in a *blame culture,* with the first *blaming* the learner and the second *blaming* the teacher (Biggs and Tang, 2011). Level 1 teaching is usually characteristic of a novice teacher and can be

categorised as unreflective. This means the teacher does not stop to consider strategies that they could adopt to make the learning more effective for the learner. As a consequence, and unless they question their practice, the learner's teaching and the learning experience is unlikely to improve (Biggs and Tang, 2011). For level 2 teaching, the responsibility for ensuring that learners actually learn now relies predominantly on the actions of the teacher. This is important as it is broadly acknowledged that effective teaching and learning should not concentrate on the mechanisms of teaching, but rather on whether or not the teaching has the required impact on the learner (Biggs and Tang, 2011). With this in mind, the third level is recognised as the most desirable, mainly as it involves combining both the learning and teaching components. At the third level, effective teaching therefore involves employing teaching strategies which encourage learners to engage with learning activities which are most likely to enable them to achieve the learning outcomes (LOs) (Biggs and Tang, 2011).

Reviewing levels 1–3, is it clear that the characteristics of level 3 are well suited to SBE, mainly as those facilitating learning must have some knowledge and understanding of the different approaches students may adopt when learning. For example, students may adopt either a surface or deep approach to learning. Surface learners usually embark on activities of a lower cognitive level than that required to achieve the LOs, and, in contrast, deep learners will undertake activities of a higher cognitive level (Biggs and Tang, 2011). The key to good teaching is to recognise that both approaches will take place, but to also recognise the importance of encouraging the most appropriate type of learning, depending on the learning situation.

Biggs and Tang (2011) present the theories of constructivism and phenomenography, both of which share the opinion that effective learning changes the way in which learners view the world. It is not just acquiring information which results in change, but rather the way in which we reflect on, and think about, this information, and build knowledge from the learning experience. Education is therefore about a conceptual change, and for this to be facilitated, four aspects to consider include:

## TABLE 3.1
### Faculty Roles, Responsibilities, and Characteristics

| Role | Responsibilities & Contributions | Characteristics |
|---|---|---|
| Coordinator | Oversees and directs the delivery of the overall session, including:<br>■ The briefing session<br>■ The simulation activity<br>■ The debriefing session<br>■ Asking learners to complete a post session evaluation | Expert faculty member<br>Well-developed organisational skills<br>Strong leadership skills<br>Excellent communication skills<br>Ability to contribute to, and lead, the development of others |
| Facilitator | The faculty member who has the most contact with the learners. This role includes:<br>■ Observing learners during the simulation activity<br>■ Guiding learner's reflection, taking them on the journey of experiential learning | Proficient faculty member<br>Focused communication skills<br>Understanding of how others learn, based on educational theory |
| Simulation Technician (ST) | Provides expert technical knowledge of simulation equipment, including:<br>■ Preprogramming scenarios on manikin software<br>■ Providing audio-visual support<br>■ Troubleshooting technical problems<br>■ Ensuring adequacy and effectiveness of equipment and consumables | Can be at any stage in the novice to expert journey and their contribution will be influenced by their level of competence<br>Solution-focused approach<br>Patience and calming influence<br>In-depth knowledge of technical equipment<br>Motivated to deliver a safe educational space<br>Focused communication skills<br>The ability to clearly articulate, and explain, technical language to the education team |
| Embedded Professional (EP) | Immersed in the simulation, their role is to insert realism to challenge and teach the learner, including:<br>Delivery of information<br>Providing prompts<br>Responding to questions to maintain the immersive situation for the learner<br>Resetting the environment, ready for the next session or clinical use | Usually, a novice or advanced beginner<br>Patience and calming influence<br>Detailed knowledge of the scenario<br>Ability to perform clinical skills (e.g., venepuncture)<br>Motivated to deliver a safe educational space<br>Focused communication skills |
| Simulated Patient | An alternative option to a manikin. Can add realism and authenticity to the simulation. Role includes:<br>Being briefed by the coordinator and using this information to help maintain the learner's immersion in the simulation<br>Delivering information and prompts, and responding appropriately to questions<br>Resetting the environment, ready for the next session or clinical use | Usually a novice<br>Patient and calming influence<br>Detailed knowledge of the scenario<br>Focused communication skills<br>Sensitive to the changing needs of the learner<br>The ability to recognise when learners are becoming overwhelmed, adapting their behaviour accordingly to maintain safety |

1. Clearly defined and transparent LOs which both facilitators and learners are aware of should be agreed.
2. Learners have a desire to achieve the LOs, and the facilitator should adopt a teaching approach designed to motivate learners.
3. Learners should be free to focus on learning without fear of unscheduled events, such as surprise assessments, as this can generate anxiety and may prevent learners' achieving deeper levels of learning.
4. A culture of collaborative working should be harnessed where learners can engage in dialogue

| | **TABLE 3.2** | |
|---|---|---|
| | **Three Levels of Thinking Relating to Teaching** | |
| **Level** | **Focus** | **Beliefs** |
| 1 | Student's characteristics and focusing on the differences between learners (good vs bad) | ■ Mostly novice teachers<br>■ Their responsibility is to know the content and present this clearly.<br>■ Teaching is transmitting information, usually by lecturing.<br>■ Curriculum is a list of content that, once presented to the learners, has been 'covered'.<br>■ Attributes differences in learning to variations in students' ability, motivation, culture, or ethnicity when students do not learn.<br>■ Ability is the main factor which determines learners' performance, and assessment is the method to measure learner's ability when teaching is finished.<br>■ Teaching is a more selective activity than an educative one, and variability in learning is founded on whether the learners are good or bad students.<br>■ When students do not learn, it is as a consequence of their failings. |
| 2 | The actions of the teacher. Priority focuses on the teacher's organisation of the learning environment, rather than the facilitation of learning | ■ Learning is viewed as a task, and focuses on what the teacher is doing, rather considering the type of learner, and their needs.<br>■ When the material to be delivered is complex for learners to understand, this requires more than chalk and talk, and work is required to attain a range of teaching skills to facilitate the delivery of material.<br>■ Teaching and learning are predominantly teacher-centred – the variety of learning activities associated with this level means the learning experience may be enjoyed by students and highly evaluated.<br>■ Focus on what the teacher is doing rather than the learning which is taking place. |
| 3 | Student-centred approach, taking account of students' characteristics and actions (student-centred) as well as the actions of the teacher, and how the student responds to these | ■ Teaching should focus on facilitation of learning, and how well students have engaged with learning.<br>■ It is unacceptable for teachers to suggest 'I taught them, but they didn't learn.'<br>■ Teaching involves becoming expert in a variety of techniques for learning, and the assessment of the success of these techniques is based on the success with which they facilitate student learning.<br>■ Teaching is more than merely a list of facts, concepts, and principles to be covered and understood by the learner.<br>■ Teaching requires clarity as to the expectations of the learner and teacher, including transparent learning outcomes, how these will be measured, and the learning and teaching strategies adopted to achieve understanding. |

Adapted from Biggs, J. and Tang, C., 2011. EBOOK: Teaching for Quality Learning at University. Berkshire, UK: McGraw-Hill Education.

with both peers and facilitators; this dialogue can stimulate deeper learning and a deeper understanding.

The levels tend to be representative of the stages in a teacher's career (Biggs and Tang, 2011). Similarly, from a simulation faculty perspective, there is a requirement to progress through these levels on the journey to becoming an effective simulation educator and reflective practitioner (Biggs and Tang, 2011).

## Experiential Learning and Reflective Practice

Within the context of SBE, learners participate, in a simulation activity, with planned intended learning objectives (ILOs), and this is followed by a facilitated debrief session. This process is an example of engaging in Kolb's experiential learning cycle (Kolb, 1984) (Fig. 3.1) in a structured and deliberate manner. Similarly, the experiential learning model described by Kolb (1984) is also the ideal approach which, through reflection and feedback, simulation faculty can develop and progress. It should be noted that novice faculty will gain the most from this process when they complete all four stages of the experiential learning cycle (Poore et al., 2014; Swanwick et al., 2019). The term 'reflective practitioner' is often associated with health and care practice; however, as facilitators of learning, it is necessary to apply these principles to our practice as simulation faculty. This is grounded in the acquisition of knowledge and creating meaning through active reflection on experiences, as well as incorporating this learning into future practice as an educator. There is also the opportunity to identify knowledge gaps and future learning needs to become an effective simulation-based educator.

In essence, SBE is a guided exercise in active reflection, with the theory of experiential learning at its core. Kolb (1984) is one of the earliest developers of modern experiential learning and describes a cycle by which learners transform real world experiences into knowledge and learning. Kolb's cycle (1984) is representative of a dynamic learning process with four elements: concrete experience, reflective observation, abstract conceptualisation, and active experimentation. Learners will develop at different rates, and have different preferred learning styles, therefore individuals will enter the cycle at the point most appropriate to them. However, learning is optimised when learners move through the cycle, rather than remaining trapped at their preferred point.

Figure 3.1 is representative of a learner's journey through the experiential learning cycle when applied to a simulation learning activity. Within the arena of SBE, the role of facilitating this process is undertaken by the faculty member facilitating the debrief.

## Miller's Pyramid for Assessment

Psychologist George Miller proposed a framework to assess clinical competence among the medical profession in 1990 (Miller, 1990). This was founded in the belief that traditional methods of medical student assessments relied heavily on testing theoretical knowledge, rather than testing its application, and the students' ability to perform in

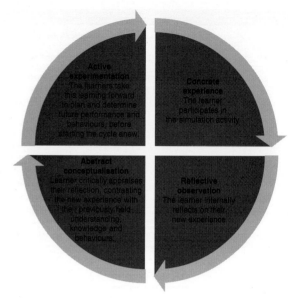

**Fig. 3.1** ■ Kolb's cycle. (Applied to learning through simulation.)

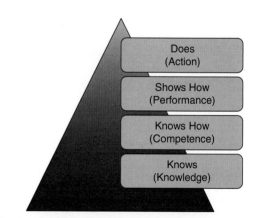

**Fig. 3.2** ■ Miller's pyramid. (From Miller, G.E. (1990) The assessment of clinical skills/competence/performance, Academic Medicine: Journal of the Association of American Medical Colleges, 65(9), pp 63–67. Adapted by Drs R. Mehay and R. Burns, UK (Jan 2009).)

practice. Miller's pyramid (Fig. 3.2) (Miller, 1990) was initially based on four levels for assessing clinical competence, with each level representative of the learning journey. Knowledge forms the foundation of the pyramid (*knows*), and as knowledge grows and understanding develops, the second level of the pyramid is reached (*knows how*), which represents application of knowledge. Ability to apply this knowledge and understanding to practice is represented as level 3 (*shows how*) which is indicative of the learner's competence in clinical skills. Lastly, clinical performance is at the top level of the pyramid. Perhaps most importantly, the lower half of the pyramid represents the cognitive attributes of competence, while the upper half corresponds to the behavioural and attributes of clinical competence.

### Mehay and Burns Prism of Clinical Competence

Mehay and Burns (2009) further developed the concept of Miller's pyramid (1990), generating a prism of clinical competence. This adaptation included a more detailed account of learner' activities and further explanation of assessment strategies which could be applied at each level. They also applied the concept of novice to expert presented by Dreyfus and Dreyfus (1980) and Benner (1982). Benner's model (1982) outlines the stages of clinical competence at different stages of career development and is widely used to assess learner's needs as they progress through their career. Finally, Mehay and Burns (2009) added the attributes of knowledge, skills, and attitudes, rendering this adapted version of the

previously created pyramid model a *prism for competence* (Fig. 3.3).

### Extending Miller's Pyramid

More recently, Ten Cate et al. (2021) extended the concept of Miller's prism and included a fifth level of 'Trusted' (Fig. 3.4). The introduction of this new level was in response to the framework of assessment of clinical competence for the medical profession which had evolved to include the concept of entrustment. Ten Cate et al. (2021) believe that the addition of 'Trusted' at the apex of the pyramid goes beyond merely performing in practice (*does*) and is representative of educators believing learners have the necessary clinical judgment skills to respond when the unpredictable happens in practice.

While Benner (1982) presented the pathway from novice to expert as a means of *measuring* competence, Miller (1994), Meahy and Burns (2009), and Ten Cate et al. (2021) instead focused on the *assessment* of competence. Although these pyramids and prisms were designed primarily to inform this assessment of clinical competence, the journey they represent at each level can in fact also align to the growth of a simulation faculty member. Similarly, the associated assessment strategies at each level are transferable to measuring the competence of the simulation educator, and Fig. 3.5 provides a visual representation of this.

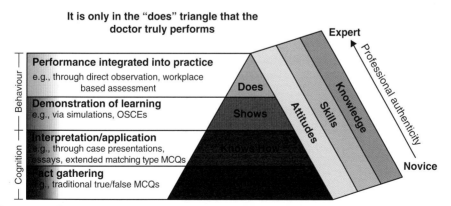

**Fig. 3.3** ■ Miller's prism of clinical competence (aka Miller's pyramid). *MCQs,* Multiple choice questions; *OSCE,* Objective Structured Clinical Exam. (Based on the work by Miller, G.E. (1990) The assessment of clinical skills/competence/performance, Academic Medicine: Journal of the Association of American Medical Colleges, 65(9), pp 63–67. Adapted by Drs R. Mehay and R. Burns, UK (Jan 2009).)

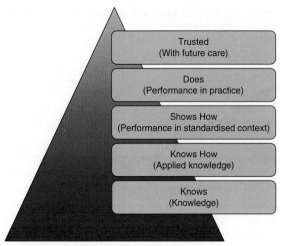

**Fig. 3.4** ■ Miller's pyramid extended. (From Ten Cate, O., Carraccio, C., Damodaran, A., Gofton, W., Hamstra, S.J., Hart, D.E., et al., 2021. Entrustment decision making: Extending Miller's pyramid. Academic Medicine, 96(2), pp.199-204.)

## APPLYING COMPETENCE PRISMS TO FACULTY DEVELOPMENT

The following section will apply the adapted prism (of simulation faculty development) to the journey of becoming a faculty member. It will provide an overview of the transition from novice to expert and becoming an autonomous simulation practitioner. Strategies for formative assessment in the context of faculty development will be presented, in recognition that this is an integral component of the journey.

### Level 1: Knows (Gaining Knowledge)

Level 1 is aligned with the novice stage. This is the beginning of the journey to becoming a faculty member and will require coaching and support from more experienced colleagues. At level 1 the normal strategy for assessment to measure competence would be written, including traditional exams and multiple-choice questions; however,

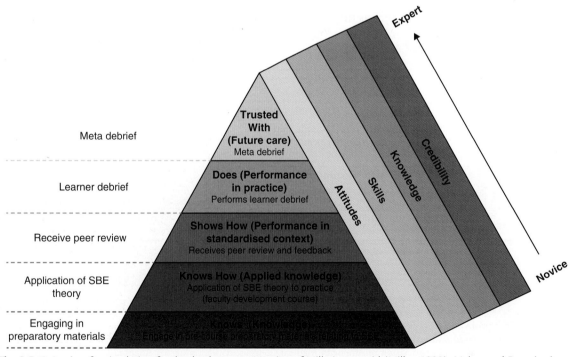

**Fig. 3.5** ■ A prism for simulation faculty development: Merging of Miller's pyramid (Miller, 1990), Mehay and Burns' prism of competence (2009), and Ten Cate's extension of Miller's pyramid (2021) aligned to the growth of a simulation faculty member. *SBE,* Simulation-based education.

in the formative assessment world of SBE, this would be measured by the completion of online learning to generate and participate in engaging discussion.

## Level 2: Knows How (Applied Knowledge)

Parallels can be drawn here with the advanced beginner stage on the novice to expert continuum (Benner, 1982). It is essential at this level to attend a faculty development course, which will present the opportunity to apply pre-course learning to a simulation session. The support of expert faculty at this level is essential to support the advanced beginner as they learn the *process* of delivering a simulation session, facilitating peer reflection, providing constructive feedback, and learning about the importance of maintaining a safe learning environment. In terms of clinical competence, the normal assessment strategy at this level would be essays or clinical problem-solving exercises. However, in SBE, competence would be assessed through practising the safe delivery of a simulation session and an associated debrief. This would be a simulated educational setting, with peers adopting the role of the learner, and experienced faculty providing feedback on the advanced beginner's performance.

## Level 3: Shows How (Performance)

This is the midway point in the journey for the simulation faculty member and aligns with Benner's *competence* level (Benner, 1982). Here, developing faculty members will demonstrate their learning by participating as part of a faculty team to deliver a standardised simulation session. They may lead the delivery of a component of the session, usually briefing or debriefing. To protect the learners and maintain the safe learning environment, an experienced faculty member should oversee this activity and they should be prepared, and able, to step in should the developing faculty member become overwhelmed. At this level, the learner progresses from assessing cognition to assessing behaviours (Miller, 1990), which would normally involve a practical element (e.g., Objective, Structured, Clinical Examination (OSCE)). This transfers to the faculty development arena as a facilitated debrief and peer review for the developing faculty member. This in turn allows for reflection and facilitates engagement in the experiential learning cycle (Kolb, 1984) as the developing faculty member grows in confidence.

## Level 4: Does (Performance in Practice)

Nearer the top of the prism, the transition from a developing faculty member to an established faculty member is well underway, and they become more proficient in managing a simulation session. A feature of this level is the ability to draw upon the valuable knowledge and skills gained, and to oversee the simulation session as a whole. At this level the faculty member should be able to adapt in response to situations, while maintaining a safe space for both learners and faculty and supporting others in the team to develop. Within the context of medical education, this level can be assessed through workplace-based assessments and direct observation (Miller, 1990), and this approach is transferable to all health and care disciplines. In terms of faculty development, the assessment of performance will be conducted by an expert colleague, using a validated debrief tool. Here, the faculty member will be formatively assessed facilitating and assessing learners undertaking a simulation activity.

## Level 5: Trusted (Demonstrates Ability to Assess Others)

The pinnacle of the prism aligns with the expert level of competence (Benner, 1982). As an expert, this faculty member will possess a wealth of knowledge and experience of SBE. Progressing from level 4, expert simulation faculty go beyond merely seeing the simulation as a whole and will intuitively anticipate problems. They will have the capacity to manage complex simulation learning activities, with an ability to deal with the unpredictable. Acting as a role model, the expert will coach and develop others, whilst having the self-awareness to recognise and plan to address their personal development needs. When faculty reflect together on their personal performance and facilitation of learning, this is known as a meta-debrief. For an expert simulation faculty member, their meta-debrief will be with peers (other experts).

## THE PROCESS OF FACULTY DEVELOPMENT

This example of a faculty development programme shares our experience and strategies for applying the principles of the prism (see Fig. 3.5). This programme is aimed at staff from all health and care disciplines who have an interest in developing as a simulation faculty member. There are two aspects to consider. Firstly, the development journey from the faculty member's perspective, which is a step-by-step approach. Secondly, planning and delivering a robust faculty development programme, underpinned by validated teaching, learning and assessment approaches (outlined in 'Teaching, Learning, and Assessment Strategies').

## Becoming a Faculty Member

Before considering embarking on a faculty development programme, we would always encourage prospective simulation faculty (regardless of their discipline) to observe a simulation course. This provides valuable insight into the individual roles and responsibilities of faculty members and the dynamics of an expert faculty team. From this initial observation, they can then make an informed choice regarding whether or not they wish to progress on the journey as a faculty member (Fig. 3.6).

The next step is to attend the faculty development course. This one-day course is predominantly practical and replicates most SBE courses. Beginning with an interactive presentation, introducing the concept of simulation as a strategy for learning, participants are orientated to the simulation environment including equipment, simulation area, control room, and support staff. After this, participants select from a bank of validated scenarios, adopting the faculty member's role to facilitate the brief, delivery, and debrief of a simulation session. After this, there is a facilitated discussion of the participant's performance, which may include recalling recorded video footage.

At the end of the faculty development day, prospective simulation faculty are supplied with a portfolio of documentation to support them through their journey, this includes (Tables 3.3–3.8):

- Simulation reflection and future objectives
- Simulation logbook
- Simulation debrief/feedback notes
- Record of simulation courses
- Non-technical skills aide memoir

After attending a one-day faculty development course, prospective faculty are invited to shadow a simulation course, preferably one which is aligned to their area of clinical expertise. To protect the safety of the learners attending the simulation session, this process for prospective faculty is gradual throughout the course of the day. Firstly, they will attend the faculty briefing meeting where they can establish their own personal goals for the day, and from this, an action plan will be developed to achieve these goals throughout their day shadowing the course. This is a necessary step to provide something tangible which they can reflect on later. They will be given the opportunity to shadow every faculty member on the day, usually beginning in the control room, before working alongside the embedded professional (EP) and being immersed in the scenario. Having observed some debrief sessions, it is anticipated that by the end of the day, they will be able to contribute to the debrief when invited by experienced faculty members.

The next stage on the journey is when the novice faculty member participates in the delivery of a simulation course. With the support of the experienced faculty, they will be responsible for the delivery of a

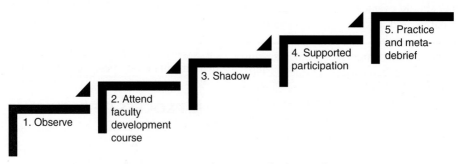

**Fig. 3.6** ■ Steps to becoming a faculty member.

| TABLE 3.3 | |
|---|---|
| **Simulation Reflection and Future Objectives** | |
| Name | |
| Date | |
| Course | |
| Scenario | |
| Co-faculty | |
| **Reflection** | |
| | |
| **Personal Take-Home Messages** | |
| | |
| **Future Objectives** | |
| | |

| TABLE 3.4 |
|---|
| **Simulation Logbook** |
| Course:........................................................... <br> Date:............................................................. <br> Level of Learners:...................................... <br> Number of Learners:.......................................... <br> Faculty:.................................................... <br> Number Debriefs:.................................... <br> Faculty Debrief: ☐Y ☐N  Lead: ☐Y ☐N |
| Personal Focus Session: |
| Scenario Challenge: |
| Debrief Challenges: |
| Learning Points: |
| Achieved Focus: ☐Y ☐N <br> Improvement/Recommendations: |
| 1. Personal: |
| 2. Course: |
| 3. Actions: |

specific element of the course, which will be agreed during the faculty brief at the beginning of the day. The supported participation stage can last for a period of time. Being cognisant that individuals will evolve and develop at a different pace, the number of courses required to move to the next stage will vary. This will only happen when they have participated in a number of courses with documented evidence of development, and when both the faculty member and their simulation mentor agree.

The final stage is reached when the faculty member is practising as a simulation team member. In addition to demonstrating that they have the essential attributes, knowledge, and skills to effectively facilitate any element of the simulation session, they will also be required to peer review and participate in a facilitated meta-debrief with their co-faculty. The meta-debrief is a quality assurance mechanism whereby faculty can reflect together on their personal performance and create action plans to facilitate further development.

| TABLE 3.5 |
| --- |
| **Simulation Debrief/Feedback Notes** |

| Scenario name: | |
| --- | --- |
| Time started: | |
| Time | Video observations |
| | |
| | |
| | |
| | |
| | |
| | |
| | |
| | |
| | |
| | |
| Comments relating to intended learning objectives/general comments | |
| | |

| TABLE 3.6 |
| --- |
| **Record of Simulation Courses** |

| Simulation Course Record | | | | | | | | | | |
| --- | --- | --- | --- | --- | --- | --- | --- | --- | --- | --- |
| Date | | | | | | | | | | |
| Course | | | | | | | | | | |
| | **Names** | | | | **Names** | | | | | |
| | | | | | | | | | | |
| | | | | | | | | | | |
| | Time | Total time allocated | Scenario | Faculty | | | | Actual time started | Actual time finished | Actual time taken |
| | | | | Agenda | Lead | Embedded Prof | Other | | | |
| 1 | | | | | | | | | | |
| 2 | | | | | | | | | | |
| 3 | | | | | | | | | | |
| 4 | | | | | | | | | | |

| TABLE 3.7 |
| --- |
| **Example of Completed Simulation Faculty Reflection Matrix** |

| Simulation Faculty Reflection | | | |
| --- | --- | --- | --- |
| Name | Facilitator 4 | | |
| Course | TEAM session medical ward | Date | 010119 |
| Scenario | Acute Asthma | Co-faculty | Facilitator 2 |
| Areas to consider | | Reflections | |
| Scenario | Scenario Management:<br>Bookmarking<br>Camera management<br>Discussion with co-faculty<br>Technical | Remember to check and cross check the recording system immediately before the scenario begins<br>Use tech support when unsure<br>Remember, becoming familiar with the recording system takes time<br>Individual discussion<br>Good teamwork with simulation technician | |
| Debrief | Agenda:<br>Reactions<br>Record verbatim<br>Limiting discussion<br>Use of questions<br>Setting agenda | Good eye contact and engagement<br>Nicely covered!<br>Good body language<br>Ask only one question at a time, then use non-verbal communication and be comfortable with silence | |
| | Analysis:<br>Use of questions<br>Use of silence<br>Use of micro teach<br>Use of video | Specific and closed questions generated good, relevant discussion<br>Important to know the local communication framework<br>Nicely framed questions and recognition of the need for micro-teach<br>Good use of stills from video to generate discussion. May consider use of video for next time.<br>Nicely concluded – remember the need to run to time | |
| | Take Forward Messages:<br>Avoid discussion<br>Record verbatim<br>Avoid validation<br>Use of questions for clarification | This is a time for clarification, and not discussion<br>Remember, it is about their learning, not yours<br>Do not paraphrase, write these down verbatim | |
| Co-facilitation | Interaction<br>Discussion<br>Support<br>Feedback | Think about hierarchy, and who makes the decisions<br>Consider using video to generate discussion and highlight learning points<br>Work with co-facilitator to confirm the plan and prevent this becoming fragmentation of discussion<br>Position yourself to be in clear view of co-facilitator, this way you will be able to see any changes in their body language which may indicated you need to interject | |
| Time management | Kept scenario to time<br>Kept debrief to time | Discuss while writing? Mixed message<br>Voice – 2/1?<br>Clarity/Agree learning before scenario begins<br>Supportive facility – clarify ------- learning<br>Clarify learning | |

| TABLE 3.8 | |
|---|---|
| **Non-Technical Skills Aide Memoir** | |
| **Skill** | **Comments** |
| **Situation Awareness**: gathering information, recognising & understanding, anticipating | |
| **Communication** strategies used, effectiveness of these: patient, team; history taking; situation, background, assessment and recommendations (SBAR) | |
| **Task Management:** planning & preparing, prioritising, providing and maintaining standards, identifying and utilising resources | |
| **Decision Making**: identifying options, balancing risks and selecting options, re-evaluating | |
| **Team Working**: coordinating activities with team, exchanging information, using authority and assertiveness, assessing | |
| **Leadership** capabilities, supporting others | |

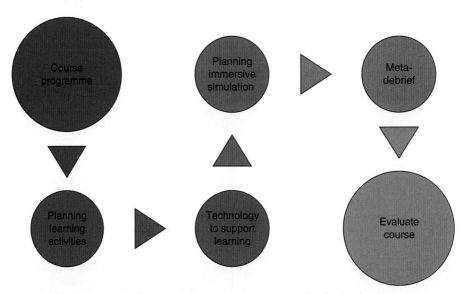

Fig. 3.7 ■ Process in planning, delivering, and evaluating a faculty development course.

## CASE STUDY 3.1: A FACULTY DEVELOPMENT COURSE

This section will share our experiences of planning, delivering, and evaluating a well-established faculty development course in the West of Scotland, which is integral to a wider faculty development programme. The overall process for this is presented diagrammatically as part of Fig. 3.7.

After completion of a faculty development course, the foundations have been established for the novice faculty member and, armed with their portfolio and supporting documents, they can begin their journey as simulation-based educators in earnest. This will include a natural progression from shadowing simulation sessions to leading on an aspect of a session. Moving forward, we will now consider the three main components in any SBE: briefing, delivering a scenario, and debriefing. The next part of this chapter will provide an overview of each of these components of a simulation course, offering guidance and some strategies for success for the novice faculty member while participating on the course.

## CASE STUDY 3.1

### A Faculty Development Course

### PLAN THE COURSE ITINERARY

This will always be the starting point, as all other activities will stem from the schedule of events planned for the day.

### PLANNING THE LEARNING ACTIVITIES

We adopt a blended learning approach, where prospective faculty receive pre-course learning materials, to promote engagement and to facilitate deep learning on the day of the course. This includes access to recordings of our team delivering a simulation brief and debrief, along with an overview of the plan for the day and information relating to their roles as they take part in the activities.

During the day the learning activities include small group discussions, planning for participating in and facilitating scenarios, and planned co-facilitation of debriefs and meta-debriefs. The ratio of course attendees (novice faculty) to faculty delivering the course is an essential consideration to optimise the novice faculty learning experience. Table 3.9 provides an overview of the course activities, and details of the documentation and equipment required for each.

### TECHNOLOGY TO SUPPORT LEARNING

To facilitate a simulation session, consideration needs to be given to the technology required for the scenario debrief and meta-debrief. It is worth remembering to enlist technical support and develop a technical equipment proforma for this (Table 3.10), to ensure parity across simulation courses.

### PLANNING FOR THE SIMULATION COMPONENT

Authenticity of consumables, and documentation reflective of current practice, is a key factor in promoting immersion in the simulation. It is worth reviewing the scenario(s) step by step to establish the requirements at each stage. An example of this can be found in Table 3.11, with a more detailed example as part of Chapter 7.

### META-DEBRIEF

The meta-debrief is the name given to the process when a debriefer is debriefed. The purpose of a meta-debrief is to facilitate faculty members' learning and development, and this is achieved through reflection and feedback. The purpose of the meta-debrief is to guide course participants by facilitating reflection to establish their thoughts on achieving their goals, and also to encourage them to consider setting goals for the future. Within the context of a faculty development course, this also provides a learning and coaching opportunity. This means time should be allowed for answering questions and, when required, to offer guidance for novice faculty (e.g., how best to transition between the stages of the debrief).

### EVALUATION OF THE COURSE

As with any learning activity, course evaluation plays a vital part in maintaining the quality of resources and delivery. It is also key if wishing to confirm that the course is enabling novice faculty to achieve the planned learning. In our experience, providing anonymity for learners who are evaluating the course reaps a more candid response, and we have achieved this in the past by promoting the use of online evaluations. These are simple to create, particularly as there are a number of online platforms which provide free tools for this purpose. Online evaluations have a number of advantages, and some have the added bonus of being able to download the results in a spreadsheet format for ease of analysis of data. Access to the evaluation can also be provided via a QR code, which can be easily generated for participants to scan using their smartphones. These codes can then be added as a part of any slide presentation, usually at the end. We prefer to 'close the loop' of the learning and teaching experienced with an evaluation, and we will often follow up the participants' post-course with a *'you said'*, *'we did'* outline when we email to thank them for attending. This approach highlights the value attributed to learner feedback, and also ensures recognition of the valuable contributions they have made throughout delivery of the course.

| **TABLE 3.9** | | |
| --- | --- | --- |
| **Course Outline with Documentation and Equipment Requirements** | | |
| Activity | Documentation | Equipment |
| 1. Introduction, housekeeping, ground rules (set the scene), ILOs and novice faculty expectations of the day | ▪ Presentation<br>▪ Copy of the timetable for the day | ▪ Projector<br>▪ Laptop<br>▪ Smartboard whiteboard/projector screen<br>▪ Paper & pens |
| 2. Interactive discussion of the SBE process:<br>▪ Pre-course materials<br>▪ Briefing<br>▪ Safe simulation<br>▪ Debriefing<br>▪ Meta-debriefing | ▪ Presentation<br>▪ Copy of the timetable for the day<br>▪ Logbook<br>▪ Reflection proforma<br>▪ Debrief feedback<br>▪ Record of course<br>▪ Non-technical skills aide memoir<br>▪ Meta-debrief tool (OSAD)<br>▪ National Simulation Educator Structure | ▪ Projector<br>▪ Laptop<br>▪ Smartboard whiteboard/projector screen<br>▪ Paper & pens |
| 3. Orientation to the simulation environment | ▪ Technical checklist<br>▪ Consumable checklist<br>▪ Clinical documentation<br>▪ Clinical guidelines | ▪ Manikins<br>▪ Clinical equipment<br>▪ Phone system |
| 4. Select scenario | ▪ Prewritten, validated scenarios | |
| 5. Practice at scenario delivery | ▪ Scenario outline<br>▪ Non-technical skills aide memoir<br>▪ Clinical documentation<br>▪ Clinical guidelines | ▪ Manikins<br>▪ Clinical equipment<br>▪ Phone system |
| 6. Practice debriefs as co-faculty (in pairs) | ▪ Board<br>▪ Pens<br>▪ Debriefing proforma<br>▪ Non-technical skills aide memoir | |
| 7. Guided meta-debrief (in pairs) | ▪ OSAD tool<br>▪ Reflection tool | |
| Repeat steps 4–7 as required based on the number of candidates | | |

*ILO,* Intended learning objectives; *OSAD,* Observational Structured Assessment of Debriefing; *SBE,* simulation-based education.

## BRIEFING

The simulation briefing is the keystone of an effective simulation learning experience. It has several aims, including orientation to the simulation environment, introductions to each other, preparation of the learners, and promotion of learner engagement. In essence, the brief allows the facilitator(s) to introduce the faculty, orientate the learners to the learning environment, and provide information required to facilitate effective learning within the simulation experience. Building an early rapport may provide insight into the learners' expectations of the course and previous experiences of simulation, enabling simulation scenarios and consequent debriefs to be adapted to the learners' needs. Although engagement can be enhanced by setting the scene and orientating the learners, it is cemented by having an open and frank discussion about the ILOs of the SBE session.

| TABLE 3.10 | |
| --- | --- |
| **Technical Equipment Proforma** | |

| Generic Technical Set Up Proforma | | |
| --- | --- | --- |
| *Date of Session* | *Candidate Numbers* | *Rooms Allocated* |
| | | |
| **Pre-Course** | | |
| | | |
| | | |
| | | |
| | | |
| **Equipment Required** | | |
| | | |
| | | |
| | | |
| | | |
| **Additional Session-Specific Requirements/Facilitator Preferences** | | |
| | | |
| | | |
| | | |
| | | |
| **Notes** | | |
| | | |

| TABLE 3.11 | |
| --- | --- |
| **Scenario Session Plan** | |

| Activity | Notes |
| --- | --- |
| Scenario:<br>10 mins maximum (1 min warning) | ■ 'Candidate' will be one of teaching faculty<br>■ Debrief will be conducted in pairs (co-facilitation)<br>■ Identify prewritten, validated scenarios to choose from, ensuring the scenario selected aligns to area of clinical expertise<br>■ Scenario brief to all candidates in classroom<br>■ Technical support will be available |
| Debrief: 20 mins approx. (2-minute warning) | ■ Using a validated debriefing tool |
| Meta-debrief: Approx. 15 minutes | ■ Led by teaching faculty<br>■ Reflective of a post-simulation debrief with candidate group as a whole<br>■ Facilitated discussion around your experience and performance during your debrief and may include video footage |

It may be that the course has predetermined ILOs, and if so, these should be communicated with the learners. As part of this, learners may be asked to generate their own ILOs and these can be documented and referenced through the subsequent debriefs and revisited at the end of the course to ensure they have been met.

The briefing session must establish a safe learning environment. The facilitator is responsible for communicating the importance of mutual respect and confidentiality to the learners as part of the brief (Cheng et al., 2014). This can be achieved in a number of ways, including asking learners to set and agree to abide by a set of 'ground rules' (Box 3.1) or asking the learners to enter into a 'fiction contract'. With the latter, learners agree to behave and react to the simulation space, and patient, as they would in their own practice environment, and therefore effectively agree to conduct themselves in a manner which would be expected of them in a professional context.

### Time Out: Ground Rules

Remember psychosocial safety is important, and this must be maintained for all participants (faculty and learners). It is always a good idea to have some strategies planned to ensure faculty have the same mental model. With this in mind, take time to consider the ground rules you would like to set and write these down.

Now consider what actions you would take in situations where ground rules have been compromised. Do not forget to include personnel and processes you may require (e.g., do you remove someone from the situation and, if so, how would you do this discreetly and safely, whilst also safeguarding all learners and faculty?).

### Orientation

It is important for novice faculty members to understand the process and sequence for orientating their learners to the simulation environment. Faculty need to be cognisant of the need to keep the orientation succinct to prevent the learners becoming cognitively overloaded in an unfamiliar environment. Time should be given to address learners' questions regarding the technical aspects of the simulation. This orientation will include:

- An overview of the equipment, including any manikins being used and the functionality of these.
- The location of any additional equipment and consumables they may require during the scenario to perform technical skills and procedures.
- An introduction to the simulation faculty team who will be involved in the session.

- Details of where learners can access additional information and resources (e.g., clinical guidelines).
- An explanation of the learner's options for seeking advice or escalating care.

---

**BOX 3.1**
## EXAMPLES OF GROUND RULES

*Psychological Safety is Where the Learners 'Feel Safe Enough to Embrace Being Uncomfortable'*
Rudolph et al., 2014.

- Simulation will highlight positive behaviour to perpetuate, as well as areas for learning and development.
- Setting realistic expectations: setting learning contract/behavioural expectations (for all).
- Inform the learners of the specific duration of the simulation and what will (and will not) happen (e.g., briefing 10 minutes; simulation 10 minutes; debriefing 30 minutes).
- Advise learners the session should stretch them and take them out of their comfort zone.
- It will be stressful but should be productive, not counterproductive (relate this to the stress curve; it should be stressful, but not counterproductive).
- If feeling stressed, please call 'Time out'.
- Be respectful and supportive of peers and faculty, avoid overly judgemental language.
- Not a test, 'What happens in simulation, stays in simulation'.
- Be prepared to ask and answer questions, be challenged.
- Allow others to speak.
- Learning space for everyone (learners and faculty).
- Phones/pagers, etc. switched to silent.
- Use of video and safety/consent.
- Treat patient and environment as real.

*Strategies to Support When Ground Rules Compromised*

- If phone rings, remind everyone these should be on silent or switched off.
- If consent not given around use of video recording, learner cannot continue on the course.
- Faculty member identified who will counsel/support anyone when required.
- Room allocated for private conversations.

---

It is always a good idea to plan the orientation in advance and to promote a standardised approach, and all key points can potentially be addressed by developing a checklist for faculty (Box 3.2).

**BOX 3.2**
## EXAMPLE OF ORIENTATION CHECKLIST

| Checklist Item | Points to Consider |
| --- | --- |
| 1. Manikin | |
| Head | Airway – can develop airway problems |
| | Head tilt/Chin lift/Jaw thrust |
| Chest | Chest movement linked to respiratory rate |
| Arms | Pulses – which ones are palpable |
| 2. Patient Monitor/Defibrillator | Describe how patient monitor works |
| | Demonstrate how to take observations with monitor |
| | Demonstrate how the defibrillator works (both automated and manual modes) |
| 3. Environment | Oxygen/suction |
| | Fluids/consumables |
| | Resuscitation trolley |
| | Telephone – call simulation switchboard |
| | Emergency kit |
| | Emergency buzzer |
| | Guidelines/British National Formulary |
| | Computer access |
| 4. Clarify Embedded Professional (EP) role | Support physical & psychological safety |
| | To give cues & keep scenario on track |
| | Able to provide information that cannot be simulated, e.g., temp, blood sugar |
| | There to help find things |
| | Communication with EP |

## THE SCENARIO

As the faculty member must have an awareness and understanding of the concept of *psychological safety*, it is important that they work towards establishing and maintaining this throughout the scenario. However, learners' psychological safety is personal to the individual and the strategy agreed as part of the ground rules. It can only be implemented if the learner decides to do this (e.g., time-out).

Novice faculty may not realise the stress felt by learners. As simulation should be a safe learning space, it is important that all faculty have an appreciation of the cognitive load felt by learners during a simulation scenario and be sensitive to signs which may indicate the learner is becoming overloaded. A spectrum of signs of cognitive overload exist and may include learner disengagement, blaming equipment, quiet learners, learners displaying anger, or learners being disrespectful. All of this is avoidable if the faculty recognises signs of overload and either changes the trajectory of the scenario or calls 'time-out', and then supports the learner to refocus.

## THE DEBRIEF

Among simulation communities, the debrief is often considered as the component where most of the learning takes place. The debrief is a facilitated learning conversation which enables learners to scrutinise their experience and simulated practice, with the purpose of developing a deeper understanding to inform the delivery of safe, effective care in future practice. The debrief may be conducted by a sole faculty member or co-facilitated by two faculty members: simulation centres around the world host faculty development courses specifically for this purpose. Good debriefing practice has the added benefit of presenting the transferable skills of active reflection on action to the learner. These are essential in the development of a culture of lifelong learning, which is required of the modern health and care professional. To fully appreciate the role of the debriefing faculty in practical terms, an understanding of the experiential learning process is required.

## Effective Debriefing

Depending on the simulation session, it may be that during a debrief there will be a time for facilitation, a time for coaching, and occasionally, a time for didactic teaching. It is important that the learning takes place in a safe environment and that learners leave the simulation safe for practice. The faculty member conducting the debrief needs to be sensitive to this and respond accordingly. In this respect, effective debriefing may require careful planning, and, without adequate preparation of the debriefing faculty, it can feel an overwhelming experience, particularly for the novice. To effectively debrief, the faculty need to be able to establish the thoughts and feelings of the learners and must be able to respond appropriately to learners' needs. By doing this, the debriefer will be able to facilitate a meaningful discussion, in a psychosocially safe way. The many facets of the effective debriefing environment include:

- Safe Learning Environment:
  - Psychosocial safety
  - Mutual respect
  - Safe space to communicate
  - Involves whole learner group
- Socratic Questions:
  - Guiding learners
  - Generate depth of discussion
  - Promote reflection on action
- Advocacy with Inquiry:
  - Technique to promote deeper learning
  - Promotes discussion
  - Establishes the underlying drivers of thought or behaviour
- Enables Reflection:
  - Active listening
  - Invite discussion
- Uses Appropriate Debriefing Strategies:
  - Use of silence by facilitator
  - Majority of talking is done by learners
  - Summarises, translating learning to the workplace

## PSYCHOLOGICAL SAFETY IN DEBRIEFING

The role of psychological safety during simulation debriefing cannot be overstated. The process of establishing psychological safety begins during the briefing session at the beginning of the simulation, and this then passes to the facilitator of the debrief to ensure it is maintained throughout the whole learning experience.

Psychological safety is the extent to which learners believe that they should take risks; it also relates to whether they believe that they will be given the benefit of the doubt (Edmondson, 2004). In essence, the group of learners must feel confident that they will not be belittled, embarrassed, or ridiculed for showing openness and vulnerability during the SBE experience; this is where the risk lies for the learner. This demands a level of mutual respect between learners and faculty.

It is common for a simulated scenario not to play out precisely the way the learner would have liked. They may, as a consequence, experience negative emotions (fear, anxiety, trepidation, and even anger) at the idea of having these events discussed and explored amongst their peers. However, this reflection and discussion of the activity which has taken place is, as we have discussed, essential for learning in simulation. These negative reactions can lead to disengagement, defensiveness, or other behaviours affecting the learner's ability to engage meaningfully in the reflective process. Usually, a negative reaction stems from previous experience. For example, learners may come from organisational environments where mistakes are viewed as the sole responsibility of the individual, and to be punished, rather than something to be explored and learned from (e.g., an environment of 'blame culture'). These reactions can have detrimental effects on other group members, evoking responses including distress, anxiety, or simply disengagement, which further negatively affects the debriefing learning process.

When learners and faculty come together to foster a psychologically safe environment for learning there is increased engagement, improved performance amongst team members, and increased learning and satisfaction amongst both learners and faculty (Frazier et al., 2017). As we explore this issue it becomes clearer that psychological safety is not something that simulation faculty can simply will into existence. Instead, this requires all group members, learners and faculty alike, to share responsibility in establishing and maintaining the psychological safety of the group. It should now be clear why maintaining psychological safety is one of the key roles of the facilitator of the debrief. With this in mind, some tactics debriefing faculty should avoid during the debrief include:

- Personal agendas: remember this is not about you; it is about the learner!
- Lengthy, personal anecdotes by the facilitator: time is precious; therefore, the focus should be on the ILOs.
- Focusing on negative behaviours as this is not characteristic of a supportive learning environment.
- Blame games or one-upmanship: this is of no benefit; the focus should be on a just culture, appreciating mistakes happen and what is important is the learning from these.
- Having a rigid and inflexible style of feedback: this does not lend itself to the adaptability required to meet the requirement of different learning styles, and learners may disengage.

## MODELS FOR DEBRIEFING

There are a number of different debriefing models available for the faculty member's toolbox, and the technique selected should be the most appropriate for the session. A number of factors may influence the choice of debriefing model, and this can depend on the simulation activity, the learners, faculty debriefer experience, or local preference. The more common techniques used are Plus-Delta, Three-Phase, and Multiphase Debriefing (Abulebda et al., 2021).

### Plus-Delta

Plus-Delta is probably the least complicated of debriefing models, where a scribe uses two columns with a (+) sign at the top of one and delta (∆) at the top of the second. The plus (+) represents the triumphs of the simulation activity, and here the scribe will document what the learners feel went well. Conversely, the delta (∆) column represents areas the learners believe were challenging, from which discussion can be generated to reach a consensus on strategies to overcome challenges in future practice. A benefit of the Plus-Delta technique is its ease of use, making it popular among novice debriefing faculty, and by its nature, it promotes easy flow of dialogue, encouraging learners to participate in discussion.

### Three-Stage Debriefing Techniques

Rudolph et al. (2006) presented one of the first three-stage debriefing models, which consisted of reaction, analysis, and summary (RAS). Since the work of Rudolph et al. (2006), a number of similar three-stage techniques have been described, including the 3D model (Defusing, Discovery and Deepening; Zigmont et al., 2011); Gather, Analyse and Summarise (GAS; Burke and Mancuso, 2012); and Diamond debriefing which involves description, analysis, and application (Jaye et al., 2015). Regardless of the specific three-stage model, Abulebda et al. (2021) present details of the common characteristics across them at each stage:

- **Stage 1** is the reaction or description stage, where facilitators should obtain the learner's true and genuine initial impressions and feelings immediately post-simulation activity. It is important to allow time for free speech from the learners and allow for their reaction without influence from the facilitator. To achieve this, allow the learners a short period of time to defuse and decompress safely, before then promoting discussion with the use of open-ended questions, to gauge learners' initial thought and feelings. Learners' initial emotional responses are validated by the debriefer who then uses the information gathered here to inform the second stage.
- **Stage 2** is the understanding and analysis stage, where facilitators use advocacy with inquiry to explore learner's appreciation of the simulation activity and their thought processes. This is where the debriefer guides the discussion to analyse the actions taken during the simulation and attempts to uncover the thought processes of the learner. From this, the debrief facilitator guides a reflective discussion with the learners to explore any gaps observed during the simulation, understand the underlying reasons for this, and collaborate to address any identified learning needs. This requires practice on the part of the debriefer, and in terms of faculty development, would be best suited to the more experienced faculty member.
- **Stage 3** is the application or summary stage, where the main points learned in the analysis stage are teased out and facilitators encourage learners to consider what they have learned, and how they plan to apply this to their future practice. Collectively, learner's 'take forward messages' are

prepared to inform either the next simulation or their health and care practice.

## Multistage Debriefing Techniques

Debriefing methods have continued to evolve as SBE has become more popular, and educational research has produced further evidence to underpin this as a strategy for learning. More recently, additional stages have been included in the debriefing process to generate in-depth, detailed dialogue for debriefing. These techniques are referred to as multistage, an example of which is the Promoting Excellence and Reflective Learning in Simulation (PEARL) model (Bajaj et al., 2018). This built on the initial three stages of the familiar RAS model, and included a fourth step where key points from the simulation could be summarised to confirm a shared mental model between the debriefer(s) and learners. PEARL is quite specific in its provision of potential word choices for debrief facilitators, and in this respect is relatively easy to use.

The role of debriefing faculty is vitally important in ensuring the learner has a positive learning experience, where they have safely consolidated some skills, and applied their knowledge of theory to their professional practice. When facilitated well, the debrief enables the learner's reflective journey. From this, learners can identify gaps in their knowledge and skills, and with the help of the facilitator, develop an action to address deficits. Faculty require specialised skills to facilitate this, emphasising the need for faculty development.

## QUALITY ASSURANCE AND THE META-DEBRIEF

Having established the significance of the debrief and the critical role it plays in learning, it is essential to preserve the quality of this component of the simulation through continuous faculty development (O'Shea et al., 2020). A strategy adopted by many simulation centres is 'debriefing the debrief' (O'Shea et al., 2020), commonly known as the meta-debrief. This quality assurance measure involves debriefers participating in regular evaluation of their practice, and receiving constructive feedback from their peers, which then informs their own focused reflections (O'Shea et al., 2020).

There are a number of approaches to the meta-debrief, ranging from one-to-one immediate feedback including end of day discussions (either one-to-one or in a group) or replaying recordings of debrief sometime later (either one-to-one or in a group).

## Evaluation Tools for the Meta-Debrief

A number of tools exist to assess faculty member's performance in the debrief. While these can be used to provide some form of quality assurance for the debrief process and learner experience, these are also a useful vehicle for developing and sustaining the skills required for effective debriefing. The most common debrief assessment tool is the OSAD (Observational Structured Assessment of Debriefing) (Runnacles et al., 2014). Albeit the OSAD is contained on one (double-sided) page, this is a detailed tool which can be used in both simulated and real health and care practice. The OSAD presents eight categories, providing a definition for each, and examples of feedback which would score low to high (Tables 3.12 and 3.13).

## CASE STUDY 3.2: CONTINUING PROFESSIONAL DEVELOPMENT

We believe facilitating the development of our simulation faculty is an organisational responsibility, and by valuing your team's commitment to your service, you can maintain and sustain a faculty to deliver SBE. As with anyone on a learning journey, faculty will develop at different rates and this may be influenced by the individual, or opportunities they may have had, or experiences they have been exposed to. Consequently, the specific skills they may wish to develop as they progress on their journey as a simulation educator can vary. In response to this, we have developed a West of Scotland approach to CPD. To date there have been a series of seven workshops developed, all taking around 4 hours to facilitate, and covering specific simulation-related topics. As time progresses, we anticipate more workshops will be developed in response to faculty requirements and changes in technology and the health and care environment. The CPD programme is designed to allow simulation faculty to select any or all of the workshops they believe would most benefit their personal needs. Staff are provided with evidence of attendance should this be required for their professional regulatory body.

A common feature across all workshops is the blended learning approach, whereby attendees are provided with self-directed pre-course reading and information and are

**TABLE 3.12**

**OSAD Categories and Definitions**

| Category | Definition | Example of a Score of 1 | Example of a Score of 5 |
|---|---|---|---|
| 1. Approach | Manner in which the facilitator conducts the debriefing session, their level of enthusiasm and positivity when appropriate, showing interest in the learners by establishing and maintaining rapport and finishing the session on an upbeat note. | 'You made lots of errors in that scenario, which is poor since I assume that you must have seen that scenario before.' | 'Let's start the session with introductions, so we can understand each other's backgrounds and previous experiences.' |
| 2. Establishes learning environment | Introduction of the simulation/learning session to the learner(s) by clarifying what is expected of them during the debriefing, emphasising ground rules of confidentiality and respect for others, and encouraging the learners to identify their own learning goals. | 'I'm not interested in what you see as the purpose of this session, but I know what I want to teach you about and it's very important to me.' | 'Please start by explaining what you hope to take away from this debriefing session. The information we discuss remains confidential.' |
| 3. Engagement of learners | Active involvement of all learners in the debriefing discussions, by asking open questions to explore their thinking. Using silence effectively to encourage their input, without the facilitator talking for most of the debriefing, to ensure that deep rather than surface learning occurs. | 'I'm now going to teach you about the correct way to do things and I'd like you all to keep quiet and listen to me.' | 'As team leader, can you describe to us what was going on at that point in the scenario? Why do you think that?' |
| 4. Reflection | Self-reflection on events that occurred in the simulation/learning session in a step-by-step factual manner. Clarifying any technical clinical issues at the start, to allow ongoing reflection from all learners throughout the analysis and application phases, linking to previous experiences. | 'I can tell you exactly what you did and why you were doing it in that way.' | 'Could you talk through what you observed, right from the start, in a step-by-step way, so we are all clear about the events that occurred?' |
| 5. Reaction | Establishing how the simulation/learning session impacted emotionally on the learners. | 'I can't understand why you are getting upset about the events in the scenario, it's never had that impact on other people.' | 'That part appeared very stressful to us observing; how did you feel at the time? Do you think that it impacted upon the rest of the experience, and in what way?' |
| 6. Analysis | Eliciting the thought processes that drove a learner's actions, using specific examples of observable behaviours, to allow the learner to make sense of the simulation/learning session events. | 'There's no point asking you why you did that, but you should know to do it differently next time.' | 'Why do you think that event happened at that particular moment? So what was distracting you then?' |
| 7. Diagnosis | Enabling the learner to identify their performance gaps and strategies for improvement, targeting only behaviours that can be changed, and thus, providing structured and objective feedback on the simulation/learning session. | 'That was all fine, I suppose, but I don't think you did anything particularly well.' | 'So you identified that your team were not aware how concerned you were; can you suggest ways in which you could communicate your concerns more clearly next time?' |

*Continued*

**TABLE 3.12 (Continued)**

**OSAD Categories and Definitions**

| Category | Definition | Example of a Score of 1 | Example of a Score of 5 |
|---|---|---|---|
| 8. Application | Summary of the learning points and strategies for improvement that have been identified by the learner(s) during the debrief, and how these could be applied to change their future health and care practice. | 'So you'll do better next time? I think you know what you did wrong in the scenario. Let's finish there.' | 'Can you summarise the key points you learnt from this session? How do you think you might change the way you manage the situation if faced with it again in your clinical workplace?' |

OSAD, Observational Structured Assessment of Debriefing.
Debriefing faculty can be scored on their performance ranking from 1 (performed very poorly) to 5 (performed very well).
From Runnacles, J., Thomas, L., Sevdalis, N., Kneebone, R., Arora, S. and Cooper, M., 2014. Development of a tool to improve performance debriefing and learning: The paediatric Objective Structured Assessment of Debriefing (OSAD) tool. Postgraduate Medical Journal, 90(1069), pp.613-621.

**TABLE 3.13**

**Objective Structured Assessment of De-briefing**

| | 1 | 2 | 3 | 4 | 5 |
|---|---|---|---|---|---|
| **1. Approach** | Confrontational, judgmental approach | | Attempts to establish rapport with the learner(s) but is either over-critical or too informal in their approach | | Establishes and maintains rapport throughout; uses a non- threatening but honest approach, creating a psychologically safe environment |
| **2. Establishes learning environment** | Unclear expectations of the learner(s); no rules for learner(s) engagement | | Explains purpose of the debriefing or learning session but does <u>not</u> clarify learner(s) expectations | | Explains purpose of debrief and clarifies expectations and objectives from the learner(s) at the start |
| **3. Engagement of Learners** | Purely didactic; facilitator doing all of the talking, and not involving passive learner(s) | | Learner(s) participates in the discussion but mostly through closed questions; facilitator not actively inviting contributions from more passive learner(s) | | Encourages participation of learner(s) through use of open-ended questions; invites learner(s) to actively contribute to discussion |
| **4. Reaction** | No acknowledgment of learner(s)'s reactions, or emotional impact of the experience | | Asks the learner(s) about their feelings but does not fully explore their reaction to the event | | Fully explores learner(s)'s reaction to the event, dealing appropriately with learner(s)'s who are unhappy |
| **5. Descriptive Reflection** | No opportunity for self-reflection; learner(s) not asked to describe what actually happened in the scenario | | Some description of events by facilitator, but with little self-reflection by learner(s) | | Encourages learner(s) to self-reflect upon what happened using a step by step approach |
| **6. Analysis** | Reasons and consequences of actions are not explored with the learner(s) | | Some exploration of reasons and consequences of actions by facilitator (but not learner(s)), but no opportunity to relate to previous experience | | Helps learner(s) to explore reasons and consequences of actions, identifying specific examples and relating to previous experience |
| **7. Diagnosis** | No feedback on clinical or teamwork skills; does not identify performance gaps or provide positive reinforcement | | Feedback provided only on clinical (technical) skills; focuses on errors and not purely on behaviours that can be changed. | | Provides objective feedback on clinical (technical) and teamwork skills; identifies positive behaviours in addition to performance gaps, specifically targeting behaviours that can be changed |
| **8. Application** | No opportunity for learner(s) to identify strategies for future improvement or to consolidate key learning points | | Some discussion of learning points and strategies for improvement but lack of application of this knowledge to future clinical practice | | Reinforces key learning points identified by learner(s) and highlights how strategies for improvement could be applied to future clinical practice |

From Arora S., Ahmed M., Sevdalis N. Evidence-based Performance Debriefing for Surgeons and Surgical teams: The Observational Structured Assessment of Debriefing tool (OSAD).

signposted to supplementary material. There are set criteria for attendance, in terms of experience, as these courses are not designed for the novice, but for those who have some experience in SBE. Each workshop has a specific lesson plan, an example of which can be found in Table 3.14.

Details of the suggested ILOs for each workshop are outlined in Case Study 3.2, and you may wish to consider these when developing your own simulation faculty and promoting ongoing CPD for faculty members.

| | TABLE 3.14 | |
|---|---|---|
| | **Example of CPD Workshop Lesson Plan (Co-Debriefing)** | |
| **Time** | **Intended Learning Objectives** | **Activity** |
| 10 minutes | Ice breaker | Introduction of faculty and participants |
| 5 minutes | Participant-derived intended learning objectives (ILOs) | Derive understanding of drivers for attendance at session |
| 15 minutes | Define relevant terminology | Definitions<br>Small group work dependent on group size or delivered directly from faculty<br>Explore participants' prior experiences of co-debriefing |
| 25 minutes | Demonstrate an understanding of the benefits and challenges of debriefing interprofessional groups of learners<br>Group work | Explore participants' prior experiences of debriefing interprofessional groups<br>Discuss concerns regarding psychological safety and re-enforcement of historical stereotypes (e.g., power imbalances, hierarchy)<br>Discuss potential for rich and meaningful learning conversations and surfacing assumptions |
| 40 minutes | Describe and analyse the benefits and challenges of interprofessional co-debriefing<br>Group work followed by review of video content | List potential benefits and challenges of interprofessional co-debriefing<br>Use video playback of case vignettes to re-enforce learning and open discussion<br>Discuss opportunities for faculty development during interprofessional co-debriefing – how is the 'meta-debrief' best conducted in this scenario? |
| 15 minutes | BREAK | |
| 30 minutes | Explore the pros, cons, and practicalities of differing co-debriefing strategies | Deconstruct 'follow-the-leader' vs. 'divide & conquer' approaches<br>Discuss potential re-enforcement of negative stereotypes<br>Work through strategy checklist items for pre-brief, pre-debriefing, debriefing, postdebriefing, and post-course |
| 20 minutes | Describe the ideal qualities of a co-debriefer | Discuss relevant differences with 'follow-the-leader' vs. 'divide & conquer' approaches |
| | Group work | |
| 10 minutes | Review session/ILOs | Describe what has been achieved and set future goals |

CPD, Continuing professional development.

## CASE STUDY 3.2

### *Workshop: Design a Simulation-Based Education Event*

Accompanying Material:
- For example, workshop slide set, flip charts & pens, high-fidelity mannikin, etc.

Prior Learning/Experience Required:
- Completion of online modules.
- Have attended a faculty development course and have some relevant experience of delivering SBE.
- Blank scenario template and example of completed scenario templates.

Intended Learning Objectives:
- Identify appropriate aims for an SBE event.
- Design SBE event taking account of stage within curricula, either undergraduate or postgraduate, uniprofessional or interprofessional.
- Design SBE event using the principles of constructive alignment.
- Consider the impact of cognitive load theory when designing SBE.

Faculty Requirements:
- Expert simulation educators, with appropriate simulation experience.

Success Criteria for Learners:
- Completion of ILOs through interaction with others within session.

*continued*

*Workshop: Non-Technical Skills Understanding and Application in Simulation Debriefs*

Accompanying Material:

- For example, workshop slide set, flip charts & pens, high-fidelity mannikin, etc.

Prior Learning/Experience Required:

- Completion of online modules.
- Have attended a faculty development course and have some relevant experience of delivering SBE.
- Suggested reading of non-technical skills (NTS) resources, for example, *Safety at the Sharp End,* and additional contemporary NTS journal articles.

Intended Learning Objectives:

- Define 'NTS'.
- Demonstrate understanding of each of the constituent components.
- Consider how NTS can be used within abstract learning conceptualisation.

Faculty Requirements:

- Expert simulation educators, with appropriate simulation experience.

Success Criteria for Learners:

- Completion of ILOs by interactivity within session.

*Workshop: Briefing - Purpose and Delivery in Simulation-Based Education*

Accompanying Material:

- For example, workshop slide set, flip charts & pens, high-fidelity mannikin, etc.

Prior Learning/Experience Required:

- Completion of online modules.
- Have attended a faculty development course and have some relevant experience of delivering SBE.

Intended Learning Objectives:

- Be able to provide a definition of 'the brief' and develop awareness of the constituent components.
- Develop awareness of the safe psychological learning environment for both participants and faculty, and how to promote this.

- Discuss the effect of mood congruent processing on learners and explore how this can be optimised.

Faculty Requirements:

- Expert simulation educators, with appropriate simulation experience.

Success Criteria for Learners:

- Completion of ILOs through interaction with others within session.

*Workshop: Making it Work – The 'Tech' and Embedded Professionals Within Simulation-Based Education*

Accompanying Material:

- For example, workshop slide set, flip charts & pens, high-fidelity mannikin, etc.

Prior Learning/Experience Required:

- Completion of online modules.
- Have attended a faculty development course and have some relevant experience of delivering SBE.

Intended Learning Objectives:

- Develop confidence with basic mannikin functionality (switching on/off, troubleshooting).
- Develop skills and knowledge in manikin functionality and operation for a scenario.
- Develop awareness of basic functionality of camera and audio-visual systems.
- Develop awareness of the skills required of an embedded professional to maintain simulation immersion.

Faculty Requirements:

- Expert simulation educators, with appropriate simulation experience.

Success Criteria for Learners:

- Completion of ILOs through practical demonstration of skills.

*Workshop: Maximising Learning Within the Debrief*

Accompanying Material:

- For example, workshop slide set, flip charts & pens, high-fidelity mannikin, etc.

Prior Learning/Experience Required:

- Completion of online modules.

- Have attended a faculty development course and have some relevant experience of delivering SBE.

Intended Learning Objectives:

- Describe underlying principles of debriefing.
- Compare contrasting strategies of debriefing for different learner groups in different settings.
- Demonstrate effective facilitation of reflective learning through debriefing skills.

Faculty Requirements:

- Expert simulation educators, with appropriate simulation experience.

Success Criteria for Learners:

- Completion of ILOs through practical demonstration of skills.

*Workshop: In-situ Simulation*

Accompanying Material:

- For example, workshop slide set, flip charts & pens, high-fidelity mannikin, etc.

Prior Learning/Experience Required:

- Completion of online modules and materials.
- Have attended a faculty development course and have some relevant experience of delivering SBE.
- Prior experience of in-situ simulation, either as participant or faculty would be beneficial.

Intended Learning Objectives:

- Define 'in-situ' simulation and explore the potential reasons for its use.
- Overview of developing a local programme for in-situ simulation.
- Explore the challenges and barriers to running in-situ simulation and explore potential solutions.
- Creating psychological safety for departmental interprofessional teams.

- Exploring the use of incorporation simulation as strategy for measuring clinical safety and quality improvement frameworks.

Faculty Requirements:

- Expert simulation educators, with appropriate simulation experience.

Success Criteria for Learners:

- Completion of ILOs through interactivity within session.

*Workshop: Co-Debriefing in Interprofessional Simulation-Based Education*

Accompanying Material:

- For example, workshop slide set, flip charts & pens, high-fidelity mannikin, etc.

Prior Learning/Experience Required:

- Completion of online modules and materials.
- Have attended a faculty development course and have some relevant experience of delivering SBE.
- Prior attendance at 'Maximising learning within the debrief' workshop.

Intended Learning Objectives:

- Define relevant terminology (debriefing, co-debriefing, interprofessional co-debriefing, interspeciality co-debriefing).
- Demonstrate an understanding of the benefits and challenges of debriefing interprofessional groups of learners.
- Describe the ideal qualities of a co-debriefer.
- Describe and analyse the benefits and challenges of interprofessional co-debriefing.
- Explore the pros, cons, and practicalities of differing co-debriefing strategies.

Faculty Requirements:

- Expert simulation educators, with appropriate simulation experience.

Success Criteria for Learners:

- Completion of ILOs through interaction with others within session.

## TOP TIPS

| Top Tip | Guidance |
|---|---|
| ■ **Psychosocial safety is paramount** | Our actions create the psychological safe space for learning. Consider the following suggestions:<br>■ Use forenames<br>■ Be honest<br>■ Be supportive<br>■ Be informative<br>■ Be timely – no one likes to rush and everyone needs a break |
| ■ **Communication is key** | Role model positive language and behaviour.<br><br>Silence can be helpful, but remember it should be framed and not awkward. No one can read your mind! |
| ■ **Simulation is a team sport** | Collaboration is key! |
| ■ **Draw on the expertise available** | Engage with subject matter experts, both practise colleagues and educators.<br><br>Every experience is a learning opportunity for faculty and learners. |
| ■ **Establish a shared mental model** | Review the event details with input from the faculty. |
| ■ **Establish debriefing rules – be specific** | It is important to agree which model/style of debriefing will be used, and to achieve consensus between faculty.<br><br>A basic set of rules for debriefing among learners establishes boundaries and clarity, i.e., 'What happens in simulation and what is said in debriefing stays here?'<br><br>Clarify the importance of active participation of learners, i.e., peer discussion enables learning, hearing others' thoughts and ideas in managing scenarios provides more tools moving forward. |

| Top Tip | Guidance |
|---|---|
| ■ **Do not forget the ILOs** | Ensure they are available/visible for everyone to review and refer to them. |
| ■ **Consider questioning style** | Open questions encourage discussion and generate more ideas.<br><br>Closed questions lead to yes/no answers and reduce opportunities for elaboration and discussion. |
| ■ **Failing to prepare is preparing to fail** | Always have a plan B! |

## SUMMARY

This chapter has explored the many facets of developing and sustaining a faculty to deliver simulation-based education. The roles and responsibilities of faculty members should now be clear, as should the importance of collaborative working among the faculty to achieve success in delivering simulation programmes. Having now provided detail of the underpinning educational theories which support SBE, and the adapted prism for simulation faculty development, it is anticipated that these processes will better enable the reader to understand and apply the development process required to become a simulation faculty member. Furthermore, the detailed account of the stages of a simulation session, and the skills required for effective simulation briefing, scenario delivery, and simulation debriefing, also provide a basis for those wishing to develop as facilitators of SBE. The need to maintain and sustain faculty has also been recognised through presentation of an overview of a regional CPD workshop. The overarching aim is that you will be able to support your own teams as they progress on their journey to becoming simulation educators. We wish you success on this journey going forward.

## REFERENCES

Abulebda, K., Auerbach, M., Limaiem, F. 2021 [Updated 2021 Oct 1]. Debriefing Techniques Utilized in Medical Simulation. In: StatPearls [Internet]. Treasure Island (FL): StatPearls Publishing; 2023 Jan. Available from: https://www.ncbi.nlm.nih.gov/books/NBK546660/

Aebersold, M., 2018. Simulation-based learning: No longer a novelty in undergraduate education. The Online Journal of Issues in Nursing 23 (2).

Bajaj, K., Meguerdichian, M., Thoma, B., Huang, S., Eppich, W., Cheng, A., 2018. The PEARLS healthcare debriefing tool. Academic Medicine 93 (2), 336.

Benner, P., 1982. From novice to expert. AJN The American Journal of Nursing 82 (3), 402–407.

Biggs, J., Tang, C., 2011. EBOOK: Teaching for Quality Learning at University. McGraw-Hill Education, Berkshire, UK.

Burke, H., Mancuso, L., 2012. Social cognitive theory, metacognition, and simulation learning in nursing education. Journal of Nursing Education 51 (10), 543–548.

Cheng, A., Eppich, W., Grant, V., Sherbino, J., Zendejas, B., Cook, D.A., 2014. Debriefing for technology-enhanced simulation: a systematic review and meta-analysis. Medical Education 48 (7), 657–666.

Decker, S., Fey, M., Sideras, S., Caballero, S., Boese, T., Franklin, A.E., et al., 2013. Standards of best practice: Simulation standard VI: The debriefing process. Clinical Simulation in Nursing 9 (6), S26–S29.

Decker, S.I., Anderson, M., Boese, T., Epps, C., McCarthy, J., Motola, I., et al., 2015. Standards of best practice: Simulation standard VIII: Simulation-enhanced interprofessional education (Sim-IPE). Clinical Simulation in Nursing 11 (6), 293–297.

Dreyfus, S.E., Dreyfus, H.L., 1980. A five-stage model of the mental activities involved in directed skill acquisition. California University Berkeley Operations Research Center.

Edmondson, A.C., 2004. Psychological safety, trust, and learning in organizations: a group-level lens. In: Kramer, R., Cook, K. (Eds.), Trust and distrust in organizations: Dilemmas and approaches. Russell Sage Foundation, New York, pp. 239–272.

Eppich, W., Cheng, A., 2015. Promoting Excellence and Reflective Learning in Simulation (PEARLS): Development and rationale for a blended approach to health care simulation debriefing. Simulation in Healthcare 10 (2), 106–115.

Franklin, A.E., Boese, T., Gloe, D., Lioce, L., Decker, S., Sando, C.R., et al., 2013. Standards of best practice: Simulation standard IV: Facilitation. Clinical Simulation in Nursing 9 (6), S19–S21.

Frazier, M.L., Fainshmidt, S., Klinger, R.L., Pezeshkan, A., Vracheva, V., 2017. Psychological safety: A meta-analytic review and extension. Personnel Psychology 70 (1), 113–165. https://doi.org/10.1111/peps.12183.

Jaye, P., Thomas, L., Reedy, G., 2015. The Diamond: A structure for simulation debrief. The Clinical Teacher 12 (3), 171–175.

Jeffries, P.R., Dreifuerst, K.T., Kardong-Edgren, S., Hayden, J., 2015. Faculty development when initiating simulation programs:

Lessons learned from the national simulation study. Journal of Nursing Regulation 5 (4), 17–23.

Kolb, D., 1984. Experiential learning: experience as the source of learning and development, 1. Prentice Hall, Hoboken.

Lateef, F., 2010. Simulation-based learning: Just like the real thing. Journal of Emergencies, Trauma, and Shock 3 (4), 348–352. https://doi.org/10.4103/0974-2700.70743.

Mehay, R., Burns, R., 2009. Miller's pyramid/prism of clinical competence. The essential handbook for GP training and education. Radcliffe Publishing, London, UK.

Miller, G.E., 1990. The assessment of clinical skills/competence/performance. Academic Medicine 65 (9), S63–67.

O'Shea, C.I., Schnieke-Kind, C., Pugh, D., Picton, E., 2020. The meta-debrief club: An effective method for debriefing your debrief. BMJ Simulation & Technology Enhanced Learning 6 (2), 118.

Poore, J., Cullen, D., Schaar, G., 2014. Simulation-based interprofessional education guided by Kolb's experiential learning theory. Clinical Simulation in Nursing 10, e241–e247. https://doi.org/10.1016/j.ecns.2014.01.004.

Rudolph, J.W., Simon, R., Dufresne, R.L., Raemer, D.B., 2006. There's no such thing as "nonjudgmental" debriefing: a theory and method for debriefing with good judgment. Simulation in Healthcare 1 (1), 49–55.

Rudolph, J.W., Raemer, D.B., Simon, R., 2014. Establishing a safe container for learning in simulation: The role of the presimulation briefing. Simulation in Healthcare 9 (6), 339–349.

Runnacles, J., Thomas, L., Sevdalis, N., Kneebone, R., Arora, S., Cooper, M., 2014. Development of a tool to improve performance debriefing and learning: The paediatric Objective Structured Assessment of Debriefing (OSAD) tool. Postgraduate Medical Journal 90 (1069), 613–621.

Sittner, B.J., Aebersold, M.L., Paige, J.B., Graham, L.L., Schram, A.P., Decker, S.I., et al., 2015. INACSL standards of best practice for simulation: Past, present, and future. Nursing Education Perspectives 36 (5), 294–298.

Swanwick, T., Forrest, K., O'Brien, B. (Eds.), 2019. Understanding medical education: Evidence, theory, and practice, 3rd edn. Wiley-Blackwell, Oxford.

Ten Cate, O., Carraccio, C., Damodaran, A., Gofton, W., Hamstra, S.J., Hart, D.E., et al., 2021. Entrustment decision making: Extending Miller's pyramid. Academic Medicine 96 (2), 199–204.

Zigmont, J.J., Kappus, L.J., Sudikoff, S.N., 2011. The 3D model of debriefing: Defusing, discovering, and deepening. Seminars in Perinatology 35 (2), 52–58.

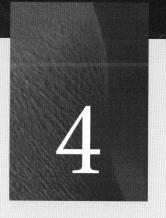

# 4

# SCENARIO WRITING FOR SIMULATION-BASED EDUCATION

ALISTAIR MAY ■ RONA KEAY

## CHAPTER OUTLINE

## OBJECTIVES

*This chapter should support the reader to:*

- Describe various ways in which simulation scenarios can be used, as an appropriate teaching and learning strategy
- Discuss an overview of educational theory which informs and underpins simulation scenario design
- Demonstrate a stepwise approach to simulation scenario design
- Discuss some of the practical considerations for simulation scenario design

Scottish Centre for Simulation and Clinical Human Factors (SCSCHF, 2022), chosen because of its efficiency and constructivist design to deliver planned learning. Throughout the chapter there are activities and examples to assist the reader to design their own scenarios.

## KEY TERMS

Scenario design

Constructivism

Fidelity

Learning objectives

Learning capacity

Embedded professional

Scenario state

Prompts

Transition trigger

Constructive alignment

## INTRODUCTION

This chapter provides an overview of simulation modalities and uses, with consideration of when and what type of simulation may be appropriate. Educational theory associated with scenario design for planned learning, mainly constructivism, is then presented. The stages of scenario design are described using the example of the method from the

## BACKGROUND

The debrief is often considered to be the key stage for learning using simulation. It provides the opportunity to reflect on the learning experience and allows the learner to consider how this will shape their future practice and enables action planning for future learning. For debriefing to positively impact on the learning experience, the process of designing a simulation activity must be robust and thorough, taking account of the desired learning, and those who will both engage with and facilitate this learning. Gaba (2007, p. 126) described simulation as '*a technique (not a technology), to replace or amplify real experiences with guided experiences, often immersive in nature, that evoke or replicate substantial aspects of the real world in a fully safe, instructive and interactive fashion.*' This description confirms the importance of scenario design and highlights how crucial this is if wishing to deliver impactful simulation-based education (SBE). The aim is therefore that, by the end of this chapter, you will have developed some understanding of why scenario design is so important when preparing to deliver an effective simulation-based activity.

## CONTEXT

The term *simulation* is broad and encompasses a variety of educational strategies and techniques. The many uses of simulation in healthcare must first be considered, mainly as the technique for writing and designing an optimal simulation will differ depending on this. Some uses of simulation include planned learning, individual, or team assessment. This could be formative (assessment *for* learning) or summative (an evaluation *of* learning against a predetermined benchmark) and systems testing (which tests processes rather than individuals). The intended use should therefore be considered as a first step when designing a scenario, or indeed whether simulation is the best strategy for what must be delivered. At this point efficiency must also be considered: resource utilisation and healthcare education costs should therefore be at the forefront when using simulation for planned learning. The scenario design approach used by the SCSCHF (see Writing Scenarios, later) will be presented in this chapter as an example of an optimal approach to simulation design to achieve planned learning.

Let's now consider some examples, beginning with formative assessment, which can occur in real clinical practice, and indeed should occur at every opportunity. Using simulation for formative assessment uses more resources than real clinical encounters. Harnessing these encounters first, before considering simulation, may avoid the need for the extra resource, or justify its use if real clinical encounters do not have suitable content for formative assessment. Every real clinical encounter could be used for formative assessment and learning, with a debrief following these real-life experiences. It is also important to recognise, however, that there is less potential to control learners' experiences in a real clinical encounter, when compared with simulation. Suffice to say, ad hoc clinical encounters limit the opportunities for planned constructivist learning, and it is the latter which is key to the success and effectiveness of SBE. Therefore, in the case of using simulation for formative assessment, you are not taking full advantage of the constructivist approach that is key to maximising the use of simulation for planned learning. As discussed later in the chapter, being able to meticulously control the activity with which learners engage (via scenario design and delivery), you will be able to create the learning you planned for them.

Simulation as a means of practising for uncommon or critical events is also useful, but first it is necessary to consider whether the simulated environment needs to be immersive to maximise effective performance in real-life. Practising some key parts in a low-tech, step-wise manner may also enable individuals to develop their competent performance. In fact, some aspects of this practise could be embedded into planned immersive simulations.

Using simulation for individual summative assessment is already taking place in the world of simulation, but perhaps this is happening out of necessity, due to lack of clinical opportunities rather than being the most effective and efficient mode of assessment. In addition, other potential issues must also be contemplated when considering simulation as a summative assessment strategy, especially issues associated with the reliability and validity of the assessment process, particularly in cases of high-stakes assessments. High-stakes assessments often generate anxiety for the learner and are considered by Dupre and Naik (2021) as those which could result in failure to progress in your role.

Simulation can also be used for assessing processes or health and care systems which, initially, may seem valid. However, if the simulation includes using a manikin in conjunction with real health and care systems, every aspect of the process needs to act and react as it would if it were a real patient going through the real system. An example of this would be using a manikin in a clinical area to test a clinical emergency response. This means despite the manikin, all resources, including equipment and staff should replicate the real world. Although you may identify some potential issues with the system, there is a risk that you will because despite best efforts, a manikin cannot replace a real person. Therefore, the information you gain, at best, reflects the work as simulated and not necessarily the 'work as done' (Shorrock and Williams, 2017, p. 124), the things that actually happen when a real patient goes through the real system (Shorrock and Williams, 2017). Depending on participants' engagement with the simulation, you may only see the 'work as imagined' (Shorrock and Williams, 2017, p. 125). This is important to recognise as simulation participants may do what they think they should be doing according to policy and protocol, and this could be very different from what actually happens in real life. This is particularly true if an analysis of the system has not been performed, pre-simulation, as there may be a variety of approaches and tools to consider (Shorrock and Williams, 2017).

There are also various combinations of resources that could be considered to be simulation. These resources may include full body manikins, simulated patients, virtual reality, or task trainers. Any one, or in fact several, of these could be used, ranging from a desktop activity in a classroom of 30 people to a fully immersive environment resembling the real-life situation. The combination of resources will depend on what you are trying to achieve for your learners. For the purposes of this chapter, we will consider 'immersive simulation'. We use this to refer to simulation built to achieve psychologically high fidelity, wherein the learners act and react in ways similar, or indeed identical, to the way they would in a real-life situation. Immersive simulation creates realistic experiences, leading to learning which can be applied to real-life situations. Although immersive simulation will be the focus of this chapter, the broad principles of designing simulation for learning apply regardless of the resources and simulation set up you decide to use.

In summary, simulation can therefore be used for each of the purposes described and this chapter will help you to gain a better understanding of why, in many situations, simulation for planned learning is the most efficient use of your resources. Establishing where and when to use simulation in your organisation is key to ensure you get the most from your resources.

### Time Out

Activity: Simulation for Planned Learning

Example: There is a new clinical pathway for patients admitted to your organisation. The pathway has been fully tested and it is now time to train the staff to help them understand and be able to use the pathway.

Think about your own area of practice. Can you identify where you could use simulation for planned learning within the context of your own area to develop your team?

## CONSTRUCTIVISM

The educational theory of constructivism forms the basis for scenario design for planned learning using simulation. Constructivism is underpinned by the belief that learning is constructed by individuals based on meaning, understanding, and experiences (Amineh and Asl, 2015). The activity that the learner engages with drives this process as they use the activity to consider their current perception and interpretation, otherwise known as their mental frames (sometimes referred to as mental model) (Fig. 4.1) (Colorado Hospital Association, 2019). The learners are then facilitated to construct new learning. In order to do this, individuals must be actively involved in the learning process to construct this new knowledge (Dennick, 2012).

Constructivism can be considered from a cognitive perspective in that learning is individualised and will be constructed on a personal basis when the learner is actively involved (Piaget, 1977). When learners encounter a situation that challenges their pre-held beliefs, such as a well-designed simulation scenario, they must engage and alter their thinking as necessary to come to a new understanding, combining this new knowledge with knowledge they already have.

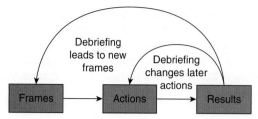

**Fig. 4.1** ■ Frames are invisible, but inferable; they are in the mind of trainees and of instructors. Actions (including speech) are observable. Most results (e.g., vital signs, order/ chaos) are also observable. (Rudolph, J.W., Simon, R., Dufresne, R.L. and Raemer, D.B., 2006. There's no such thing as "nonjudgmental" debriefing: a theory and method for debriefing with good judgment. Simulation in healthcare, 1(1), pp.49-55.)

From a social perspective, new constructs are created through interaction with others (Vygotsky, 1986), and this is then integrated with existing knowledge. This interaction may occur within a simulated scenario as well as during the debriefing conversation. The debrief offers an opportunity to facilitate learners to construct new knowledge and learning. During the debrief, exploration of learner mental frames can occur through discussion, guided by the facilitator.

When thinking about simulation scenario design, and the constructivist principle that adults construct their own learning based on their own experiences, it is possible to shape learning by carefully designing and controlling the activity that learners engage with, at each stage of the scenario. Furthermore, if the simulated activity is directed in such a way that it includes all of the building blocks for the planned learning, when it comes to debriefing, learners will begin constructing their learning as intended, as soon as the debrief begins. Therefore, constructivist learning around your intended learning objectives will happen if your scenario is carefully designed and controlled to deliver those objectives. In order to be immersive, the learner has to be unaware of this behind-the-scenes guidance and it must appear real to them when they interact with it. Taking account of this, scenario design is an important first step towards achieving the appropriate and planned learning during the debrief.

## Constructive Alignment

The principles of constructive alignment have been described by Biggs and Tang (2011). They suggest that learning will be maximal if the learning outcomes (LOs), learning activities, and assessment methods are aligned. Although it is recognised that in scenario design for learning, we are not assessing learners in the truest sense, take-home messages at the end of a debrief can be used to determine whether constructive alignment has been achieved (Fig. 4.2). Asking the learners what they are going to take away (home) from the session allows you to assess whether or not the LOs have been achieved and what learning has been gained. In reality, this is also an assessment of the faculty in terms of the success of delivering the learning that was planned. If the scenario design is robust, it has been driven as planned, and the debrief has been successful, the take-home messages should reflect the LOs. If the take-home messages consistently do not match the LOs, it could be worth considering whether or not the scenario should be altered. At this stage it may also be useful to question which part, if any, of your process is not working. Figure 4.2 provides a diagrammatic representation of constructive alignment in action as part of scenario design.

## INTENDED LEARNING OBJECTIVES

The first step in designing any simulation activity is to determine the intended learning objectives (ILOs). ILOs are statements which clearly define what you aim for the learner to know or be able to do following a

**Constructive alignment**

Scenario is built on learning objectives

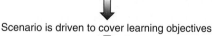

Scenario is driven to cover learning objectives

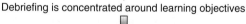

Debriefing is concentrated around learning objectives

⬇

THMs mirror the learning objectives

**Fig. 4.2** ■ Constructive alignment in simulation for learning. *THMs,* Take-home messages. (Reproduced with kind permission from the Scottish Centre for Simulation and Human Factors.)

learning event (Kennedy, 2006). It is important to recognise that there is a difference between ILOs and LOs:

- ILOs are the learning you set out to deliver
- LOs measure the learning that has actually taken place

Language is a marker of ethos here; if you truly subscribe to constructivism as an approach to simulation for learning, only ILOs can be set, and the actual LOs will only be evident if you look for them after the event. This therefore becomes an assessment of the educator, and their reflections on whether or not they managed to help learners achieve the outcomes expected when setting out the ILOs.

To create ILOs, the facilitator is required to know the learner's level of knowledge and experience. It is also important to know why the simulation activity is being created because this will inform the design of a scenario which will be relevant to the learner. Undergraduate or professional curricula may be a starting point for identifying required learning. For example, when designing a new course, it may be worth inviting learners to collaborate in the process. By inviting them to complete a questionnaire, we would be able to establish their learning priorities, making the scenarios learner driven. An alternative strategy may include scoping the workplace to establish learning needs. This could involve understanding service requirements, looking at service developments, or analysing data from significant adverse events. These are events which merit investigation to reduce the likelihood of future patient harm (Flin, O'Connor, Crichton, 2017). It is important to consider whether immersive simulation is the most appropriate learning tool for that particular learning to occur, particularly because of its potential cost in terms of resources.

The principles of scenario design apply to any type of learning content, but immersive simulation provides a platform for non-technical skills (NTS) training (Bennet et al., 2021). Immersive simulation provides a vehicle for NTS to be learned and practised in an authentic, realistic environment and provides an opportunity for learners to practise real behaviours. Planned scenario design offers the opportunity to create learning for specific NTS. Behavioural markers which are observed non-technical behaviours are at the core of NTS. Examples of behavioural categories which can be observed include situational awareness, leadership, communication, or teamwork (Yule et al., 2006). There are many resources available in the field of NTS, and as with any education, you must be well-read with a deep understanding of the subject matter before embarking on educating within this field.

You may be tempted to design a scenario around multiple ILOs, and this is understandable and likely driven by a desire to maximise learning opportunities. However, when using immersive simulation for learning in a planned way, it is particularly important to limit the ILOs in number and ensure that the scenario material is carefully and deliberately crafted to deliver the ILOs in the debriefing phase. Each ILO will correspond to a discrete part of the scenario; therefore careful consideration should be given to the number and focus of these. Once ILOs are written, these can be used as building blocks to design the scenario. The learning of NTS is complex and requires both time and cognitive effort on the part of participants, and when writing ILOs, you should remember that learning will be completed at the end of the debriefing, rather than immediately following the scenario, and almost certainly never within the immersive stage. It is useful to write ILOs in the format of *'By the end of the scenario and debriefing, learners will be able to…'* (Box 4.1). The scenario has to be authentic to maintain credibility and support learner engagement. In simulation for planned learning, it is a privilege to be able to write and direct a learning experience that has the balance of realism while avoiding extraneous complexities and focuses on planned ILOs.

---

**BOX 4.1**
### INTENDED LEARNING OBJECTIVES APPLIED TO BLOOM'S TAXONOMY

*Intended Learning Objectives*

'By the end of the scenario and debriefing, learners will be able to…'.

- Recognise a non-ST elevation myocardial infarction (NSTEMI) **(Apply)**
- Apply current guidelines for the treatment of NSTEMI **(Apply)**
- Demonstrate ability to effectively and appropriately delegate tasks **(Apply)**
- Demonstrate effective communication skills in a dynamic clinical situation **(Analyse)**

## Time Out

Using the template provided, list ILOs for your selected learners. Please remember, ILOs should be Specific, Measurable, Achievable, Realistic, Time Sensitive (SMART), and appropriate according to the level of the learner. Consider:

- What do I want the learner to know or be able to do following the scenario?
- Is my ILO specific – do I know exactly what I want the learner to know?
- Can the learner do this already? (If so, it is not an ILO!)
- Is simulation the best learning modality for this ILO?
- If I use simulation to deliver learning for this ILO, will the learner leave the simulation activity with new knowledge?

When considering the level of learner, the verbs associated with Bloom's Taxonomy of learning (Bloom, 1956) should be adopted (Table 4.1). This educational approach is designed to guide the learner incrementally from lower-order to higher-order levels of thinking. This should be based on the learner's level of knowledge and experience, beginning with a base level, before progressing to analysis, and eventually evaluation levels of thinking.

## CAPACITY TO LEARN

Capacity for learning within immersive simulation is complex and can be influenced by multiple factors, including cognitive capacity, challenge, stress, and emotion. To use the well-established Yerkes and Dodson (1908) law, humans experiencing the optimum amount of pressure will perform optimally. The stress curve is indicative of this.

This almost certainly reflects the degree of mental engagement and cognitive capacity at the time. For an intellectually challenging environment, in simple terms, the brain needs to be activated enough, but not overloaded. It follows that the ability to learn is affected by the amount of pressure felt by the learner. Within the context of simulation, this is dependent on the level of difficulty and familiarity with the planned activity. Guadagnoli and Lee (2004) described the challenge point framework for maximal retentive learning with respect to psychomotor tasks, recognising this requires a careful balance in terms of challenge. Dewey (1938) stated that learning is most effective when learners are in a state of uncertainty, as this creates a need to investigate strategies to resolve the situation. Relating this to scenario design for

| TABLE 4.1 | |
|---|---|
| **Taxonomy Level and Intended Learning Objectives Verbs** | |
| Levels of understanding (Bloom's Taxonomy) | Intended learning objectives verbs which can be applied to your scenario design |
| 1. Remembering | Identify<br>Define<br>Recall |
| 2. Understanding | Explain<br>Describe<br>Discuss<br>Reflect |
| 3. Applying | Practice<br>Implement<br>Demonstrate |
| 4. Analysing | Distinguish<br>Deconstruct<br>Integrate<br>Inquire |
| 5. Evaluating | Prioritise<br>Assess |
| 6. Creating | Develop<br>Build (on previous knowledge) |

learning in immersive simulation, the scenario could be written to have content which forces the learner slightly out of their comfort zone and allows them to question their existing knowledge and develop new understanding.

In terms of emotions, Sargeant et al. (2008) found that negative emotions can interfere with receiving effective feedback, and Seabrook (2004) suggested that students feeling embarrassed or intimidated may be unable to discuss their experiences or ask questions. Rogers et al. (2019) have found that, in simulation, there are both more positive and negative emotions displayed by scenario participants in contrast to observers. Although they did not find a direct link between emotions and learning in their study, previous research with simulation has shown a link between strong emotion and motivation to learn (Pekrun, 2006).

In terms of learning through simulation, we have established that a degree of stress is essential. Moderate levels of stress can lead to improved learning retention, particularly if the stress is related to the learning task. However, if the stress is related to an extraneous source, such as emotions or memory, retention can be detrimentally affected, decreasing the learner's capacity to learn clinical skills (Fraser et al. 2012; LeBlanc, 2009).

Psychological safety is another important factor which is key to effective learning in simulation. This must be considered when determining an appropriate stress level for your participants. A psychologically safe learning environment is one in which learners feel that risks can be taken without threat of negative consequence (Edmondson, 1999). You can use the actions of learners to underpin the learning conversation within the debrief. While psychological safety should be established during briefing at the beginning of your session, it is essential to maintain this throughout the entire session (Rudolph et al., 2014).

In summary, the learners' experience throughout the simulation process, from the moment they walk through the door to the moment debriefing finishes, is key. There needs to be enough challenge to engage the brain, but excessive pressure or challenge has a detrimental impact on learning and psychological safety. Challenge should

therefore ideally arise from realistically engaging with the activity itself (the briefing, the scenario and debriefing) and not from extraneous factors. We can now hopefully see that these principles are embedded in the construction of an immersive simulation activity.

## FIDELITY AND SCENARIO DESIGN

Fidelity should be considered during scenario design, as learner engagement can be affected by the degree of perceived reality. It is now clear that, in simulation, fidelity is not an 'all or nothing' concept, but a spectrum, and can be considered to have various facets. Rudolph et al. (2007) presents a simplified set of three ways in which humans think about reality: physical, conceptual, and emotional, which is in keeping with the levels of fidelity described.

- **Physical fidelity** refers to the realism generated when performing a skill and using the equipment. An example could be when checking a radial pulse, and the realistic nature of the manikin's skin and pulse.
- **Conceptual fidelity** refers to the authenticity of the presenting case, and response to actions by the learner. For example, you would expect to see documented evidence on a vital signs chart of hypotension in a patient with hypovolaemia; therefore if the patient is hypertensive, this will not fit with the clinical picture. This lack of attention to detail can compromise the immersion of the learner in the simulation.
- **Emotional fidelity** refers to the realism felt by the learner through their participation in the simulation. For example, the stress encountered by the learner when recognising and managing a patient with an acute asthma exacerbation.

We will now think specifically about creating a scenario for simulation, and the application of these characteristics. The physical aspect relates to the realism of the simulation, and how this looks, sounds, and feels. For example: Does the face look real? Are the heart sounds realistic? Can you feel pulses in the correct place? Is the environment authentic (is the patient on the correct bed or trolley)? For the purposes of scenario design, we consider how closely to reality the simulation acts and reacts. For example, when atropine is administered to the manikin, does the heart rate speed up? And if so, over what length of time?

The emotional facet is perhaps one of the reasons why immersive simulation can be so powerful. This is the degree to which learners are physically present and psychologically engaged in the scenario and can determine learner's response to events. By following a logical approach to the simulation, learners can then relate this to real-life behaviours and performance.

For scenario writing, consideration should be given to how important the various types of fidelity are in order to meet your ILOs. Depending on the type of simulated learning event, it may be important to prioritise one form of fidelity over others. This means presenting signs and symptoms exhibited by the manikin should reflect the classic presentation of a patient with that condition, and adjuncts to patient assessment, such as observation charts, should reflect contemporary practice. When the ILOs are in the NTS domain, emotional fidelity (the realism felt by the learner) becomes more important. However, all aspects of fidelity should be optimised to achieve an immersive state.

The model presented by Rudolph et al. (2007) (Fig. 4.3) illustrates how the three modes of fidelity combined can create realism within the scenario, which serves to increase learner engagement. The learner is then more likely to behave as they would in real life, in turn offering an opportunity for experiential learning which they can apply to their practice.

The level of fidelity which is achievable may, however, be determined by the available equipment. For example, if the focus of the ILO is technical skills, such as learning a procedural skill, physical fidelity will be more of a priority than emotional fidelity. Regardless of the type of fidelity, the 'fiction contract' should be established with learners at the beginning of the session. A fiction contract is an explicit acceptance that elements of the scenario may not be realistic due to practical considerations.

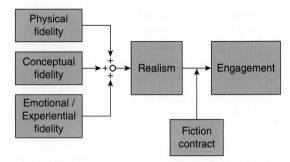

**Fig. 4.3** ■ Modes of fidelity in simulation which can contribute to increased realism and scenario engagement. (From Rudolph, J.W., Simon, R., Raemer, D.B., 2007. Which reality matters? Questions on the path to high engagement in healthcare simulation. Simulation in Healthcare, 2(3), 161-163.)

An example of this may be when a real person is adopting the role of the patient, you may choose to use a cannulation arm for venepuncture, as part of the scenario. By acknowledging this from the outset, you can separate and isolate any unrealistic aspects, to maximise learner engagement with the parts that are realistic.

### Time Out

- What elements of your simulation scenario need to be high fidelity to achieve this ILO?
- What resources do you have?
- Are there any elements that could be lower fidelity without affecting the learning?

### Example

ILO: Demonstrate effective team briefing with respect to negotiation and allocation of individual roles.

To achieve this all we need is a team of people (learners), a reason for them to form a team (e.g., a standby call), enough baseline information, and time to allow them to allocate roles. In terms of level of simulation equipment fidelity, this could be considered low. What is important is the learners need to believe that the patient will arrive at the clinical area they will be in. You should be able to achieve a high conceptual and emotional fidelity.

## Embedded Professional: Enabling Fidelity

The embedded professional (EP) (Boyer and Mitchell, 2020) has been defined as:

*'An individual who is trained or scripted to play a role in a simulation encounter to guide the scenario and might be known or unknown to the participants; guidance may be positive or negative, or a distractor based on the objectives, level of the participants, and the needs of the scenario' (Lioce, 2020, p. 16).*

The EP is pivotal to scenario authenticity and progression. Detailed briefing of the EP before the session begins is essential to ensure they are familiar with the level of learner (to achieve emotional fidelity), the scenario and initial state (physical fidelity), and any triggers for transition (conceptual fidelity) (Fig. 4.4). Some centres operate a control room from which teaching faculty can communicate with the EP via an earpiece to ensure the scenario progresses to achieve the ILOs. However, in centres with no control room, a line of communication between teaching faculty and the EP must be established. An example may be an EP leaving the scenario to collect blood bottles, but in fact using this as an opportunity to communicate with the teaching faculty.

In terms of scenario design the EP's role must fit with the situation, and realistically reflect practice (conceptual fidelity). For example, the EP acting as a hospital porter will not be able to prepare and administer intravenous fluids or check medications with a nurse in the scenario. If these tasks are intended to be part of the scenario, and to promote fidelity, the role

---

**Synopsis: Stuart Watkins CHI: 12072544**
 49-year-old male with Non-ST elevation myocardial infarction (NSTEMI).

**Patient set up**
Male patient. Awake in hospital gown, cannulated and sitting upright in bed.
Nurse present. Care pathway, Medication prescription chart and early warning score (NEWS 2) chart available.

**Information for the learner(s)**
Paged by nurse [EP]

S. It's the nurse here from the receiving unit. We have a 49-year-old male experiencing acute chest pain
B. He was seen in the emergency department for chest pain but had no ECG changes.
Transferred to medical unit and awaiting a 6-hour troponin blood test
A. He has more chest pain now.
R. Can you come and see him please?

**ABCDE – Initial state**

Airway
Airway patent – complaining of central, crushing chest pain
Breathing
Respiratory Rate 20, SpO$_2$ 95% on air, 97% on O$_2$, Lung fields clear
Circulation
Heart rate 90 regular (Normal sinus rhythm), Blood pressure 130/85, Capillary refill time 2 secs,
Skin temperature – normal, Urine output – not measured, no signs of bleeding,
complaining of central chest pain, 12 lead ECG shows T-wave elevation anterior leads.
Disability
ACVPU: Alert, Glasgow coma scale 15: E=4, V=5, M=6, Blood glucose monitoring 6.4
Exposure
No abnormalities detected, Temperature 37.1°C

**Fig. 4.4 ■** Example of brief for embedded professionals.

of the EP may need to be altered, and the tasks redesigned, or removed, from the scenario.

### Time Out: Use the Template to Draft a Brief for Your Embedded Professional

| |
|---|
| **Synopsis: Patient name and unique patient identifier** |
| **Patient set up:** |
| **Information for the learner(s):** (use your local communication handover tool, e.g., Situation, Background, Assessment, Recommendation (SBAR) or Reason, Story, Vital Signs, Plan (RSVP)) |
| **ABCDE – Initial State**<br><br>Airway<br><br>Breathing<br><br>Circulation<br><br>Disability<br><br>Exposure |

## WRITING SCENARIOS

Once the ILOs, the capacity to learn in terms of challenge, the fidelity, and the role of the EP have been considered, the scenario can now be constructed. It is essential that all elements of the scenario are documented clearly to enable members of faculty to deliver the scenario effectively. Use of a template enables a consistent approach and ensuring version control of each updated version allows changes to be discussed and agreed as the scenario is developed.

There are various scenario templates available to assist in developing and structuring the scenario. The SCSCHF Scenario Storyboard Tool is one example (Tables 4.2 and 4.3). This template is specifically designed for writing actively driven, constructively aligned scenarios to deliver planned learning through facilitated debriefing. The scenario is separated into 'states' with each state corresponding to an individual ILO. Recalling the principles of constructivism, each driven state of the scenario provides material to inform the learning conversation during the scenario debrief.

### Transition Trigger

The first thing to consider for each state is the event which must happen to signify that the learners will be able to construct the learning you plan within the debrief. Generally, the transition trigger is something that learners do or say which confirms their thought processes at this state in the scenario. When writing a scenario, it can

| TABLE 4.2 | | | | |
|---|---|---|---|---|
| **The Scottish Centre for Simulation and Clinical Human Factors Scenario Storyboard Tool** | | | | |
| **Scenario Storyboard** | | | | |
| **State name** | **State** | **Desired learner behaviours and triggers to move to next state** | | |
| **Intended Learning Objective (ILO) 1** | **Patient Response** Physiology Other Events | **Learner Actions** *May happen* *May not* *Not essential* | **Transition Trigger** (Action) *The one learner action that must happen* *Aligned to ILO*<br><br>**Prompts** Physiology *Subtle* Patient response *Realistic!* Faculty *Realistic!!* | **Additional Teaching Points** Things to cover in debriefing over and above the ILO associated to the state |

| TABLE 4.3 |
|---|
| **Example of Completed Scenario Template** |

| Scenario Storyboard | | | | |
|---|---|---|---|---|
| **State name** | **State** | **Desired learner behaviours and triggers to move to next state** | | |
| **Initial State** Thorough clinical assessment | **Airway** Airway patent (complaining of central, crushing chest pain) **Breathing** RR 20 SpO$_2$ 95% air, 97% on O$_2$ Lung fields clear **Circulation** HR 90 reg (NSR) BP 130/85 CRT 2 secs Skin Temp – normal Urine Output – not measured No signs of bleeding Complaining of central chest pain 12 lead ECG ST elevation lateral leads **Disability** ACVPU Alert GCS 15:E4, V5, M6 Blood Glucose = 6.4 **Exposure** No Abnormalities Temp 37.1°C | **Learner Actions** A to E Assessment Recognises Acute Coronary Syndrome (ACS) +/- O$_2$ Morphine Nitrates Aspirin Lower Molecular Weight Heparin Beta Blocker | **Transition Trigger** Diagnoses ACS and initiate treatment **Prompts** Physiology 12 lead ECG ST segment elevation lateral leads Patient response Alert Orientated Chest Pain 10/10 Faculty If slow to recognise ACS nurse will prompt | **Additional Teaching Points** ■ NICE Guidelines (NG185) ■ Task delegation ■ Team communication ■ O$_2$ Therapy |

ACS, Acute coronary syndrome; ACVPU, patient response – alert, new confusion, voice, pressure, unresponsive; BP, blood pressure; CRT, capillary refill time; ECG, electrocardiogram; GCS, Glasgow coma scale; HR, heart rate; RR, respiratory rate; SpO$_2$, peripheral oxygen saturation; ST, ST segment of ECG.

be challenging to specify the transition trigger because it relies on the learner having an awareness of the necessary steps required to progress the scenario. For example, in Table 4.3 there is a reliance on the learner to recognise acute coronary syndrome and treat this according to guidelines. This suggests the learner has appreciated the focus points of the scenario, which will facilitate discussion relating to the ILOs during the debrief. If this fails to happen, the EP can provide prompts to direct the scenario at this state. If this does not happen, it will become more difficult to capture intended learning during the facilitated debrief. Overall, the deeper learners think within the scenario state, the more fruitful the debriefing conversation will be. Once your transition trigger has been achieved, you generally will move on to the next scenario state and, therefore, the next ILO.

## Time out: Create a Transition Trigger for Your Intended Learning Objectives

- Ensure the transition trigger and ILO are well aligned. It is worth remembering that you need the ILO to be brought up for discussion in the debrief.
- Do not be so specific that the transition trigger is unrealistic to reach.
- Do not be so vague that the transition trigger does not prompt desired discussion during the debrief.

ILO: Recognise a non-ST elevation myocardial infarction (NSTEMI)

Example of transition trigger: Diagnose ACS

## State

Once the transition trigger has been identified, you can begin to craft the state to drive the learners towards progressing the scenario. Every piece of information that you include in the state will shape what the learners do and, more importantly, what they start to think about. The patient will respond, physiology will change, and certain events will occur in a very specific way that both reacts realistically to what is occurring and also drives the learners towards the transition trigger. It is useful to ensure that patient characteristics are documented and clear in your scenario state to guarantee the same events and learning each time that scenario is delivered. Once you get experience in this method of scenario design, you will realise that you can add various features to the scenario which will provide the material to embark on your debrief for planned learning. It is also useful to take time to think about how the patient state will result in your transition trigger. For example, if your transition trigger is 'any oxygen applied to patient', an initial high oxygen saturation is likely to drive the learner away from the transition trigger because they may allow the patient to continue breathing room air. Conversely, extremely low oxygen saturation may over-challenge them and again drive them away from the transition trigger as they desperately attempt to get help, forgetting to apply oxygen. Although the transition trigger is a clear line on your storyboard, the way the scenario moves from one state to the next needs to remain realistic in terms of conceptual fidelity to maintain immersion. For example, in a real patient, oxygen saturations will physiologically take time to increase in response to oxygen therapy, and the transition from one state to the next in your scenario must appear realistic.

## Learner Actions

Learner actions are the things that you predict *might* happen. Whether they do happen or not is irrelevant to the learning you plan, but rather a barometer of whether your scenario is being delivered as you require. Predicting in advance what people might do allows you to detect when things are moving off the track required. In terms of immersion, predicting what learners may or may not do allows preparation and mitigation for aspects that might interfere with immersion. For example, if you have a manikin without venous access

functionality, but obtaining venous access would realistically occur, you can design that out of the scenario. The EP can be very useful for these situations by realistically appearing to do the things that cannot be done by learners in a realistic way. Even more fundamentally, is there a plausible reason why the manikin may already have venous access? In rare situations where it would break immersion for someone other than the learner to perform the task, because in normal circumstances it would be the learner, consider how to do this in the most realistic way possible in order to keep the learners immersed. In this example, you could perhaps replace the manikin arm with a cannulation arm.

## Prompts

Now that you are versed in a constructivist approach, you will realise that, irrespective of the learner's action or inaction, the transition trigger must occur, otherwise there will not be the required material for the debrief. This is where the concept of prompts is required. A prompt is something that is used to move the scenario state towards the transition trigger. It is important to accept that, as long as the material is present in the scenario, immersion is maintained, and the learners have noticed, it does not matter how the material gets there. If the transition trigger is 'any oxygen applied to the patient', it does not matter who ultimately applies that oxygen, including the EP. Any prompts required need to be available, realistic, and embedded within the state to ensure that immersion is not disturbed. Prompts can come in many forms and may include something the simulated patient says or does, physiology changes, or other things in the environment, such as a telephone call orchestrated by other faculty members, or faculty entering as another member of staff to help. Prompts can be fed in via the EP in the form of comments, questions, or actions. The EP is at most risk of breaking the immersion bubble at these points, and much care must be taken in the interaction with the learners to prevent this. The EP comments, questions, and actions all need to be realistic within the situation, and this will ensure that a scenario state can be *prompted* forwards without breaking immersion. Ultimately, the EP can produce the material for you, for example, by performing the transition trigger themselves. However, if this is the case, you may need to consider redesigning your scenario state to ensure learners reach the transition triggers with less prompting. Ideally, prompts should be planned in advance and recorded on the scenario storyboard, although in practice you will often see effective ways to prompt the first few times you deliver a new scenario. In the perfectly designed scenario, prompts are not required; however, in practice, these are used to keep the scenario on track and progress to the next state. If learners are spending scenario time doing things that are not aligned to either the transition triggers (and therefore the ILOs) or to engagement and immersion, it may be worth considering changes to ILOs.

## Time Out: Prompts (Table 4.3)

| Prompts |
|---|
| Think about what pieces of information you can use to drive your participants towards the transition trigger. Consider:<br>• Having multiple prompts prepared – you never know exactly what your participants are going to do.<br>• Having prepared prompts from different sources, e.g., patient observations, embedded professional, manikin voice.<br>• Grading your prompts from most subtle to most strong, allowing adaptation during the scenario depending on participant actions. |

| Template | Example | Your template |
|---|---|---|
| **Transition Trigger:** (Action) *The one learner action that must happen* *Aligned to LO* | **Transition Trigger:** | **Transition Trigger:** (Action) |
| **Prompts:** Physiology *Subtle* | **Prompts:** Physiology | **Prompts:** Physiology |
| Patient response *Realistic!* | Patient response | Patient response |
| Faculty *Realistic!!* | Faculty | Faculty |

## TOP TIPS

| Top Tip | Guidance |
|---|---|
| • **Think about the purpose of the scenario and make this a priority** | When designing a scenario, it is essential to appreciate why immersive simulation is being used – so consider why.<br><br>Is the experience aligned to curricula? If yes, which and why? And is this the best option?<br><br>These considerations are important as immersive simulation can be expensive. |
| • **Consider what it is that you want to achieve** | Think about the planned learning and how you can best design ILOs which align with this. |
| • **Remember that detail is essential** | It takes time and subject expertise to write a scenario.<br><br>It also requires testing and changing based on evidence and practice to ensure the necessary detail is provided as part of the scenario. |
| • **Remember to evaluate the scenario to enable improvements** | Does the scenario work? Consider take-home messages of learners and whether these reflect the ILOs.<br><br>And remember – very rarely will your first draft be the perfect scenario. |
| • **Remember to liaise with and involve the faculty** | Discuss the scenario with subject experts and education faculty as this will help you to ensure that it is realistic and authentic. |

## SUMMARY

Remember, scenario design is not a singular event. You will need to spend time initially creating a scenario with transition triggers, states, actions, and prompts that you *think* will work to deliver your planned learning in the debrief. However, until that scenario is actually delivered to your target learners, it will be impossible to predict exactly how successful it will be, and if your ILOs will be achieved during debrief. It is okay if your scenario does not go exactly to plan first time. Once you gain proficiency with this technique, you will find your scenarios are very effective during first delivery. Observe, take notes, and think about what changes you can make for the next time you deliver the scenario. This applies to everyone at any level of experience in scenario design, and can also apply to well-established scenarios if, for example, there has been a change in clinical guidelines since the scenario was initially written. Therefore, if you manage to achieve the perfect scenario, congratulations! But it may be that your scenario development is ongoing and remains a work in progress.

Finally, the significance of scenario design for achieving planned learning in SBE is hopefully now clear. Meticulous creation of ILOs, and the subsequent scenario design to achieve these, facilitates planned learning during the debrief. The scenario should be actively driven via the use of transition triggers and prompts to match the ILOs and underpinned by the principles of constructive alignment. The learner's take home messages will then be more likely to align with the ILOs following the debrief. With this at the fore, we hope this chapter has given you some insight into the application of educational theory to scenario design, and that you feel equipped with the skills and tools required to successfully design an immersive simulation scenario.

## REFERENCES

Amineh, R.J., Asl, H.D., 2015. Review of constructivism and social constructivism. Journal of Social Sciences, Literature and Languages 1 (1), 9–16.

Bennett, R., Mehmed, N., Williams, B., 2021. Non-technical skills in paramedicine: A scoping review. Nursing & Health Sciences 23 (1), 40–52.

Bloom, B.S., Engelhart, M.D., Furst, E.J., Hill, W.H., Krathwohl, D.R. (1956). Taxonomy of educational objectives: The classification of educational goals. Vol. Handbook I: Cognitive domain. New York: David McKay Company.

Boyer, T.J., Mitchell, S.A., 2020. Utilization of embedded simulation personnel in medical simulation. In: StatPearls [Internet]. StatPearls Publishing, Treasure Island, (FL).

Biggs, J., Tang, C., 2011. Teaching for Quality Learning at University. McGraw-Hill.

Colorado Hospital Association, 2019. Understanding learner's frames (mental models). [online]. Available at: https://cha.com/wp-content/uploads/2019/04/3.5-Understanding-a-Learners-Frames-Mental-Models.pdf.

Dennick, R., 2012. Twelve tips for incorporating educational theory into teaching practices. Medical Teacher 34 (8), 618–624.

Dewey, J., 1938. Logic - The Theory of Inquiry. Henry Holt and Company, New York.

Dupre, J., Naik, V.N., 2021. The role of simulation in high-stakes assessment. BJA Education 21 (4), 148–153.

Edmondson, A., 1999. Psychological safety and learning behavior in work teams. Administrative Science Quarterly 44 (2), 350–383.

Flin, R., O'Connor, P., Crichton, M., 2017. Safety at the Sharp End: A Guide to Non-Technical Skills. CRC Press, Boca Raton, Florida.

Fraser, K., Ma, I., Teteris, E., Baxter, H., Wright, B., McLaughlin, K., 2012. Emotion, cognitive load and learning outcomes during simulation training. Medical Education 46 (11), 1055–1062.

Gaba, D.M., 2007. The future vision of simulation in healthcare. Simulation in Healthcare 2 (2), 126–135.

Guadagnoli, M.A., Lee, T.D., 2004. Challenge point: a framework for conceptualizing the effects of various practice conditions in motor learning. Journal of Motor Behavior 36 (2), 212–224.

Kennedy, D., 2006. Writing and Using Learning Outcomes: A Practical Guide. University College Cork, Cork, Ireland.

LeBlanc, V.R., 2009. The effects of acute stress on performance: implications for health professions education. Academic Medicine 84 (10), S25–S33.

Lioce, L., 2020. Healthcare simulation dictionary. In: Society for Simulation in Healthcare, second ed. Agency for Healthcare Research and Quality, Rockville, MD.

Pekrun, R., 2006. The control-value theory of achievement emotions: Assumptions, corollaries, and implications for educational research and practice. Educational Psychology Review 18 (4), 315–341.

Piaget, J., 1977. Intellectual evolution from adolescence to adulthood. Cambridge University Press, Cambridge.

Rogers, T., Andler, C., O'Brien, B., van Schaik, S., 2019. Self-reported emotions in simulation-based learning: active participants vs. observers. Simulation in Healthcare 14 (3), 140–145.

Rudolph, J.W., Simon, R., Dufresne, R.L., Raemer, D.B., 2006. There's no such thing as "nonjudgmental" debriefing: a theory and method for debriefing with good judgment. Simulation in Healthcare 1 (1), 49–55.

Rudolph, J.W., Simon, R., Raemer, D.B., 2007. Which reality matters? Questions on the path to high engagement in healthcare simulation. Simulation in Healthcare 2 (3), 161–163.

Rudolph, J.W., Raemer, D.B., Simon, R., 2014. Establishing a safe container for learning in simulation: The role of the presimulation briefing. Simulation in Healthcare 9 (6), 339–349.

Seabrook, M.A., 2004. Clinical students' initial reports of the educational climate in a single medical school. Medical Education 38 (6), 659–669.

Sargeant, J., Mann, K., Sinclair, D., Van der Vleuten, C., Metsemakers, J., 2008. Understanding the influence of emotions and reflection upon multi-source feedback acceptance and use. Advances in Health Sciences Education 13 (3), 275–288.

Scottish Centre for Simulation and Clinical Human Factors, 2022. NHS Forth Valley. [online]. Available at: https://scschf.org/ Accessed August 2022.

Shorrock, S., Williams, C., 2017. Human Factors and Ergonomics in Practice. CRC Press, Boca Raton, Florida.

Vygotsky, L.S., 1986. Thought and language (Rev. ed. / translation revised and edited by Alex Kozulin. ed.). MIT Press, Cambridge, MA.

Yerkes, R.M., Dodson, J.D., 1908. The relation of strength of stimulus to rapidity of habit-formation. Journal of Comparative Neurology and Psychology 18 (5), 459–482.

Yule, S., Flin, R., Paterson-Brown, S., Maran, N., Rowley, D., 2006. Development of a rating system for surgeons' non-technical skills. Medical Education 40 (11), 1098–1104.

# 5

# SIMULATION FOR SKILLS ACQUISITION

NEIL McGOWAN ■ NICHOLAS HOLT ■ KATH SHARP

## CHAPTER OUTLINE

## OBJECTIVES

*This chapter should support the reader to develop an understanding of the:*

- Strategies required to set up practical skills teaching sessions
- Rationale for adopting an evidence-based approach to practical skills teaching
- Construction of a practical skills session plan
- Teaching methods that begin a pathway to mastery of learning
- Importance of reflecting on teaching sessions to implement improvements using one suggested evidence-based method
- Integration of practical skills teaching sessions as an adjunct to healthcare education

## KEY TERMS

**Practical skills teaching**

**Low fidelity simulation**

**Part task trainers**

**Small group teaching**

**Large group teaching**

**Deliberate practice**

**Reflective practice**

**Mastery of learning**

**Constructive feedback**

**Four-step approach to skills teaching**

## INTRODUCTION

Within a healthcare environment, the term 'practical skills' covers an array of clinical examination and intervention techniques which are used to evaluate and treat patients. Skills can range from completing routine observations, such as measuring and monitoring blood pressure, oxygen saturations or range of movement, to more complex interventions, including the insertion of a central venous catheter or the emergency surgical repair of a ruptured aortic aneurysm. The level of competence in performing these skills can result in a range of clinical consequences that may impact on patient safety.

Due to the variety of practical skills health and care practitioners require, it is very difficult to describe in detail how best to learn, attain, evaluate, and maintain each singular skill. This chapter will therefore aim to present how best to plan, teach, and evaluate acquisition of practical skills, based on educational theory, using low-fidelity task trainers. The focus will also be on strategies for teaching practical skills commonly encountered by health and care practitioners.

## BACKGROUND

The term 'clinical' is derived from the Greek *klinikos* which has been defined as pertaining to or around the sick bed. Clinical skills and basic examinations were first developed around 2000 BCE, by the ancient Egyptians and Ayurvedic practitioners. These basic skills were subsequently further developed around the time of Hippocrates (450 BCE) and then Galen (CE 200), where the concept of using the five senses to get to a diagnosis emerged. The basic clinical skills in use today have in fact changed very little since the development of formal medical education programmes in Europe and North America back in the 19th century. With the advancements in technology, however, we have seen the evolvement of other practical skills to complement our diagnostic and treatment processes.

Historically, clinical skills teaching adopted an apprenticeship style approach and was delivered at the patient's bedside, with further small and large group teaching in the classroom and lecture theatre. This was apt for the time, in the absence of formalised curricula, objective evaluation, or the feedback and reflection that exists today, as the core of health and care education programmes.

Over the past 50 years, clinical procedures and investigations have changed significantly as a consequence of technological developments. Previously, patients were often talked about, or over, rather than talked to or with, and the guiding principle of Halsted's 'see one, do one, teach one' model (Kotsis and Chung, 2013) was not always the easiest (or safest) method for the patient. This was still in place as little as 20 years ago. The 'see one, do one, teach one' ideology was accepted in clinical practice as the norm when caring for real-life patients. Here, a healthcare student or newly qualified practitioner watched a procedure, attempted the next one, and then often went on to supervise another colleague or student during the next attempt at the procedure. No standardised method of

teaching, evaluating, or reflecting on the abilities of learners existed, and feedback was only received when the senior healthcare practitioner criticised the learner for making a mistake. The past 20 years have seen a changing clinical environment and working practices. There has also been the introduction of 'clinical skills laboratories' because no patient, student, or healthcare practitioner should be exposed to the risks of this archaic method of teaching practical skill acquisition in the 21st century.

## CONTEXT

With the advances in technology and clinical practice, practical skills are an integral part of daily work life within the health and care setting. These skills need to be learned to assess and treat patients in our care. The evolution of how these skills are taught, however, has been slow, with the potential for associated risks to patient safety.

There is no singular optimal method for teaching practical skills, as their range is wide and the learner group variable. The gold standard would be to align the teaching of a skill to the learner group. Which practical skills should be taught, and to which learner group, are important considerations, mainly as expectations vary across disciplines. For example, the General Medical Council (GMC) of the United Kingdom (UK) has stipulated in the outcomes for graduates that all newly qualified doctors should be proficient in a wide range of skills that are expected of a doctor (General Medical Council, 2018). The Joint Royal College of Physicians training board (2019) has a curriculum which postgraduate doctors should address as part of their training to progress. Similarly, the Nursing and Midwifery Council (NMC) (2018) and the Health Care Professions Council (HCPC) (2022) have skills standards, both for preregistration health and care education, and also for those wishing to practice in more advanced clinical roles. Therefore, the learning needs of the learner group can be both specific and very different.

### The Role of Simulation in Practical Skill Acquisition

Changes in health and care education have resulted in a move away from the traditional apprenticeship model being accepted as the process for skills acquisition

(Egan and Jaye, 2009; Mann, 2011). Instead, over the last 20 to 30 years, simulation has become an essential part of the process by which skills are acquired, supporting the growth of clinical skills training (Maran and Glavin, 2003). Historical and contemporary literature suggests that newly qualified practitioners struggle with practical skills acquisition due to either a lack of exposure or limited opportunities to gain appropriate experience during their training (Burford, Whittle & Vance, 2014; Illing et al., 2013; Monrouxe et al., 2018; O'Sullivan and Jeavons, 2005; Simpson, 2004; Williams, Leong & Gill, 2013). Simulation therefore offers learning opportunities which can complement real-life clinical experience. Early exposure to skills, using a simulation-based approach, also allows learners to commence a path to mastery throughout their subsequent training. For some professions, newly qualified practitioners may be required to be competent in a skills laboratory setting before being permitted to practice on patients. Even through more advanced stages of postgraduate training, patient safety is appropriately at the heart of all skills undertaken. Trainees should therefore not be undertaking skills they have not first practiced in the skills laboratory, and then carried out under the supervision of a practitioner who is competent in that skill. A much more structured approach was therefore recognised as being required (Egan and Jaye, 2009; Mann, 2011).

Aligned with this, it is pertinent to recognise that simulated learning environments can be deemed as low, medium, and high fidelity. In terms of simulators for skills teaching, an example of low fidelity could involve a task trainer such as a venepuncture and cannulation arm or a urinary catheterisation model. Medium- or high-fidelity simulators are often preprogrammed, computer-driven manikins, to allow display of physiological and pharmacological parameters, enabling replication of real patient interactions. Whilst it is relevant to recognise differing levels of fidelity, a meta-analysis (Kim et al., 2016) concluded that while different levels of simulation environment have educational benefits for learners, the impact of the simulation on the learner is not related to the fidelity. What is important is that all simulation sessions for skills acquisition are at an appropriate level for all learners, ensuring that it will address the intended learning objectives (ILOs) of the session and enable learners to achieve the desired learning.

## THE THEORY OF TEACHING A SKILL

Learning within health and care education is underpinned by adult learning theory, which recognises the importance of the collective influence and interaction of all actively engaged learners within the learning environment (Lave and Wenger, 1991; Mann, 2011). A community of practice is defined as the participation of a group of learners involved in a learning activity (Lave and Wenger, 1991). In this respect, learners become active participants, learning from, with and alongside all of the community members (Egan and Jaye, 2009; Mann, 2011). Each learner contributes their own personal knowledge, sharing previous experiences and practical abilities and, through dynamic interaction with the group, a sense of self-efficacy in their ability to perform the skill is developed (Bandura, 1986; Mann, 2011). Learners emulate, or become, role-models, initiating the development of personal professional identities (Mann, 2011).

Although this chapter concerns 'practical skill acquisition', this cannot, and should not, be viewed in isolation. The indications, risks, and benefits for any procedure may come under the domain of clinical reasoning and clinical decision making, but they are interwoven within the practical skill itself, and therefore should also be considered within the theory of skills teaching.

When teaching a skill, the aim is to improve the competence of the person undertaking the skill. This may be a health and care student learning a skill for the first time, such as the insertion of a peripheral venous cannula, or a senior practitioner looking to perfect central venous cannulation. Stuart Dreyfus and Hubert Dreyfus first described a five-stage skills acquisition model in 1980, when working with the US Air Force (Dreyfus and Dreyfus, 1980). The Dreyfus model sees learners develop from novice to expert as they practice and become more familiar with the rules, features, and procedural steps of a skill. Five levels were described as part of the Dreyfus model (Fig. 5.1).

### Mastery-Based Learning

Across health and care professions, a number of frameworks exist to support and develop practical skills. One method of teaching practical skills which has become increasingly popular is mastery-based learning (also discussed in Chapter 4). This involves sustained, deliberate practice with reflection, and timely constructive,

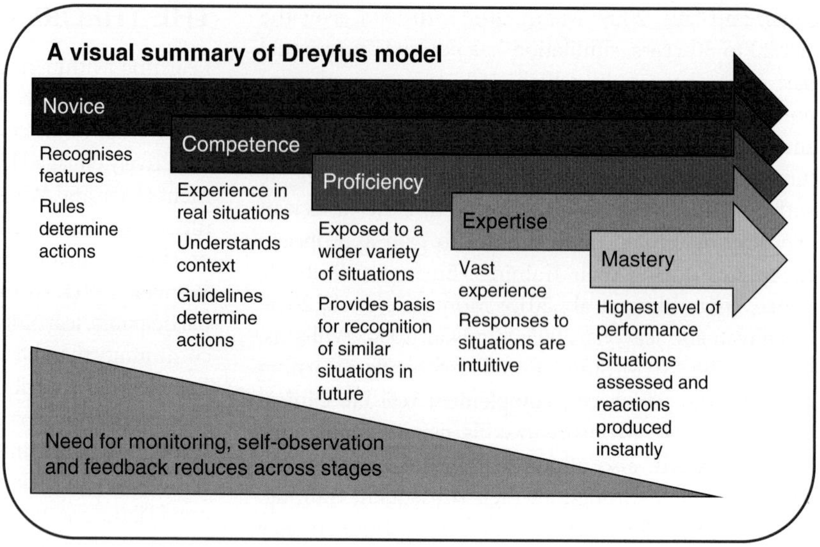

**A visual summary of Dreyfus model**

**Fig. 5.1** ■ The Dreyfus model. (Image obtained from https://richrtesting.com/the-dreyfus-model-a-visual-summary/)

feedback to take the learner on the journey from novice status to, over time, that of mastery.

It is well documented that experience and innate ability alone do not produce experts (Ericsson, 2004; Issenberg et al., 2002). Rather, it is the deliberate and repetitive performance of skills in a focused environment, with specific and constructive feedback, that allows the development of expertise (Ericsson, 2004; Ericsson, Krampe, & Teschromer, 1993; Ericsson and Lehman, 1996; Issenberg et al., 2002). However, improvements in skills performance can be short-term, and the risk of skill atrophy has been reported as potentially occurring within a 6-month period (McGuire et al., 1964). Therefore, one simulation session is often not sufficient, and simulation should be used as an adjunct to complement ongoing clinical practice to develop expertise.

Sustained deliberate practice on task-trainers offers highly valuable learning opportunities where novice learners acquire skills transferable to clinical practice in a mistake-forgiving environment (Ericsson, 2004; Issenberg et al., 2002; Kruatter et al., 2015; Wayne et al., 2006; Ziv, Ben-David & Ziv, 2005). It has been found that deliberate practice, integrated into a curriculum with clear ILOs, dramatically increases the skills of learners (Wayne et al., 2006) and begins the path towards mastery of the procedure (Issenberg et al., 2002; Issenberg et al., 2005; Nikendei et al., 2005).

In reference to the Dreyfus model, and the five levels, a mastery approach should take the learner

from novice to competent within the simulated environment. Practically, this should mean that all practitioners are at the same minimum standard before undertaking supervised practice within the clinical environment (McGaghie, 2020). In practical terms, as part of this process, this could be achieved as follows:

1. A list of essential steps is generated by experts within the field and translated into a checklist format.
2. The procedure is recorded in an audio-visual format for learners to view preprocedure.
3. Learners then perform the procedure with an experienced facilitator observing, marking off the steps on the checklist as this is carried out.
4. There is facilitator–learner reflection at the end of the procedure. If all elements have not been achieved, the process is repeated until attainment of all elements of the checklist.
5. Peer to peer marking can also occur as a formative learning process prior to a summative assessment.

## Clinical Reasoning and Clinical Decision Making

Simulation and skills laboratory teaching can also be used to develop clinical reasoning. Clinical reasoning and decision making is the healthcare professional's ability to assess a patient, analyse the gathered data accurately to identify the problem, and subsequently make decisions based on that information (Higgs and

Jones, 2008; Murphy, 2004). For learners to grow and thrive in a fast-paced, dynamic health and care system, they require high-level clinical reasoning skills to safely and effectively manage patients with complex care needs within pressured time constraints (Ericsson, 2007; Murphy 2004). Through practice and feedback, professionals can develop and progress their clinical reasoning and decision-making skills from novice to expert levels (Ericsson, 2007; Murphy 2004). However, learners continue to require a sound core knowledge base in order to make reasoned clinical decisions (Chamberland et al., 2015; Norman, 2005). In simple terms, practitioners, over time, develop two pathways of thinking: analytical and non-analytical. These will often overlap, and clinicians will move between the two depending on the situation (Croskerry, 2009).

## PLANNING

Before embarking on any plan for the delivery of a skills teaching session, there are several essential considerations including the location and what physical space is necessary, the provision of equipment (both static and consumables), personnel required, and the learning needs of learners.

### Location

Venues for skills teaching in health and care can range from the acute clinical or care environment to a dedicated training facility. Both have benefits and drawbacks. Using an off-site facility provides a physically and psychologically protected space where learning cannot be interrupted by clinical pressures. However, time taken to travel to venues can reduce time available for teaching and learning.

If using a facility on-site within the clinical or work environment, it is imperative this is a protected space. Makeshift skills teaching areas, such as overflow or apparently unused clinical areas, can be remobilised at short notice and your well-planned session could easily be cancelled due to lack of venue. Ideally, there should be adequate lighting, handwashing facilities, and adequate storage space, especially if planning to use makeshift teaching areas.

It is important to distinguish, at this point, between skills teaching and in-situ simulation, the latter of which is discussed in Chapter 6. As the purpose of in situ simulation is to allow the application of practical skills, and measurement of your systems and processes within the context of the clinical environment, the location for these sessions has to be the physical clinical or work environment.

### Time out

Take time to think about the area you will be using for your skills teaching session. Write down:
1. Where is it?
2. What is good about the area and what challenges might you encounter?
3. What facilities do you have in the area, and how can these be adapted for your session?
4. How many people can the environment facilitate (including teaching faculty)? This will give you an idea of your maximum class size.

### Equipment

This is essential. It is important to remember that low-fidelity manikins and task trainers can be just as, or even more, effective than their high-fidelity counterparts. The decision of which to use will depend on various factors, including what you have available, faculty competence in its use, the skill you are teaching, and the needs of the learners.

### Fidelity

With respect to healthcare simulation, fidelity has been described as 'the extent to which the appearance and behaviour of the simulator/simulation matches the appearance and behaviour of the simulated system' (Maran and Glavin, 2003, p. 23). This fidelity can be graded by level as low, medium, and high.

#### Levels of Fidelity Explained

An example of low-fidelity simulation would be a task trainer (e.g., an arm for venepuncture or peripheral venous cannulation). As the lowest level fidelity, and least realistic, the purpose is to allow initial practice of a skill and build learner confidence. Low-fidelity simulation is useful for single skill acquisition.

An example of medium-fidelity simulation would be a full-body manikin, which would allow a more complex clinical examination. These manikins tend to have additional functionality which can include breath sounds, heart sounds, and bowel sounds. This is useful when bringing skills together for a more detailed patient assessment and can help to build learners' cognition.

An example of high-fidelity simulation would be a full-body manikin with the highest levels of functionality, or a simulated patient (real person). These manikins, or real people, are useful for conducting physical assessments and making clinical decisions according to the findings. For the manikin, the associated computer hardware can be used to simulate patient monitors, allowing for real-time response to treatment. This is useful for developing learners' clinical reasoning skills.

Before undertaking any teaching session, a list must be constructed of the essential equipment required and any props required. It is beneficial to develop a checklist, that can be added to, or checked each time a session is delivered. It should reflect all of the equipment that is used within normal clinical settings to maximise the realism of the procedure. It is a good idea to think through the skill you will be teaching step by step, including pre-skill stages such as consent and hand hygiene, to the point of completion. By taking this approach, you will be able to identify the equipment you will need from beginning to end. Refer to Table 5.1 which uses the example of a local procedure for arterial blood gas (ABG) sampling and how the procedure informs the equipment list. This strategy can be used for fundamental to advanced skills.

## Time Out

Consider the skill you plan to teach and create a procedural checklist, noting the equipment you will require at each step of the procedure.

| TABLE 5.1 | |
|---|---|
| **Equipment List** | |
| **Preparation** | |
| Gathers equipment with minimal assistance:<br>▪ PPE<br>▪ Skin cleanser<br>▪ Arterial blood gas (ABG) syringe<br>▪ Dry swabs<br>▪ Sharps disposal | ▪ Gloves, apron, appropriate face mask<br>▪ Alcohol 70%<br>▪ Heparinised ABG syringe with needle and cap<br>▪ Non-sterile gauze swab<br>▪ Small sharps disposal box with lid |
| Introduces self & confirms patient identity | **No equipment required** |
| Explains the procedure to check there are no contraindications and gain consent | **No equipment required** |
| Undertakes modified Allen's test<br>▪ Ask patient to make closed fist, occlude both radial and ulnar arteries; patient opens palm which should be pale; release ulnar artery and then time duration for palm reperfusions (normal <5s); repeat for radial artery. | **No equipment required** |
| **Procedure** | |
| Performs hand hygiene | Hand washing facilities, liquid soap, single-use paper towels, foot pedalled disposal bin with lid, appropriate bin liner |
| Puts on appropriate-sized gloves | Non-sterile gloves sizes small, medium & large |
| Positions patient's wrist | Part task trainer<br>Chair for patient |
| Cleanses area with skin cleanser | 70% alcohol or chlorhexidine 2% wipe |
| Offers local anaesthetic, checking for allergies | Topical anaesthetic with dressing |
| Checks if ABG syringe requires air to be expelled and does this | Heparinised ABG syringe with needle and cap |
| Re-palpates radial artery with non-dominant index and middle finger, proximal to point of intended needle insertion | **No new equipment required** |
| Inserts ABG needle and syringe at 30–45 degree angle, immediately below fingers into the point of pulsation | **No new equipment required** |

| TABLE 5.1 (Continued) | |
|---|---|
| **Equipment List** | |
| Awaits flashback of blood into ABG syringe | Red stained fluid to replicate arterial blood sample |
| Holds syringe still, does not pull back on plunger | **No new equipment required** |
| Achieves adequate sample of at least 1 mL | **No new equipment required** |
| Withdraws needle steadily and immediately applies pressure to puncture site using non-sterile gauze | Non-sterile gauze |
| *Post-Procedure* | |
| Ensures pressure applied to the area for min 3 mins | **No new equipment required** |
| Removes needle from syringe and expels air | **No new equipment required** |
| Applies cap to end of syringe | **No new equipment required** |
| Safely disposes of sharps in sharps box | **No new equipment required** |
| Gently inverts syringe to ensure heparin mixed through | **No new equipment required** |
| Labels sample with patient's details | Pre-printed patient labels |
| Prepares to send sample for analysis in correct receptacle | Sample collection bag, lab forms, lab system access |
| Arranges for analysis, documenting FiO$_2$ & temperature | Patient vital signs chart |
| Documents procedure | Patient notes |
| *General Considerations* | |
| Maintained communication with patient | **No equipment required** |
| Smooth transition between procedural steps | **No equipment required** |
| Aseptic non-touch technique maintained throughout | **No equipment required** |

## Faculty

The success of any simulation session relies on a cohesive faculty to plan, deliver, and evaluate the session. This means not only those delivering the education, but those responsible for administration, coordination, and technical support. Each of these key personnel play a role essential for the delivery of a clinical skills programme, and they must be part of the team from the outset. Depending on your organisation, having an individual assigned to each of these roles may be a luxury. It may be that you need to adopt more than one (or all) role(s) in the planning, delivery and evaluation of your skills session. Nevertheless, this can help you draw up a 'to do list' for your sessions.

### Administrator

Essential to any teaching programme is the identification of someone to take on the role of administrator. Ideally, this will be a dedicated person, employed for this specific role, but in some organisations, this role needs to be undertaken by the educator or education team. If this is the case, it is worthwhile remembering this aspect takes time, and you will need to factor this into your planning stage.

The administrator role includes organising advertisement of courses, fielding queries, booking both learners and faculty for the session and, if they are aware of the appropriate teacher to learner ratio, ensuring that this is not exceeded.

You may be planning an element of pre-course learning, which can range from reading to podcasts. The dissemination of this, the session schedule, location of session, directions to the venue, distribution of any pre-course assessment, post-course evaluation and collation, and reporting of these, all fall under the remit of an administrator. Additionally, you may be in a position where you are competing for access to facilities and a venue, and an administrator can help coordinate and secure booking of a venue.

## Technicians

As the world of simulation expands at an exponential rate, so does the range and scope of equipment. From low-fidelity venepuncture arms to high-fidelity mannequins, a working knowledge of set-up, functionality, maintenance, and troubleshooting is required. The role of simulation technician has developed over the last 15 years and is now an integral part of any teaching faculty. However, not all simulation centres are fortunate enough to have technical support, and as a simulation educator, you have a responsibility to ensure you, or a member of the teaching faculty, are able to set up, operate, and troubleshoot equipment.

## Facilitators

Facilitators for skills-based teaching require to be credible, experienced, and competent in the field they are teaching. Because this teaching is based on knowledge of a skill, and the ability to teach using simulation, and does not focus on the individual's professional identity, cross-professional teaching can occur. This mix of skill and experience enriches the learning environment and is often referred to as co-facilitation. An example of this could be teaching peripheral venous cannulation, a skill undertaken by a number of different professions. In this respect a nurse could teach it to a paramedic, but only a paramedic colleague with expertise in the field can contextualise the skill for the paramedic learner.

Lastly, facilitators need to be attuned to the learner's capacity to learn (see Chapter 4, section Intended Learning Objectives). An awareness of external pressures, whether real or perceived, need to be considered, alongside the direct effects of these on the learner's emotional relationship with the learning process. For example, if acquisition of a practical skill is viewed as a 'pass/fail' component of a qualification, there will be associated psychological stress. This stress will influence the learning process. Sensitivity to this and a knowledge of strategies to manage it are essential skills for all facilitators if capacity to learn is to be optimised.

## Time out

Table 5.2 provides an example of the activities required to plan, deliver, and evaluate a simulation session for the delivery of practical skills. Use this template to note what you think you will need for a session you are organising. Also note who will be responsible for each part of your to do list, alongside a timeframe for completion.

| TABLE 5.2 | | |
|---|---|---|
| **Example of Faculty Roles and Responsibilities** | | |
| **To Do** | **Responsible** | **Timeframe** |
| Write intended learning objectives and lesson plan | Educator | 3 months pre-session |
| Develop pre-course materials:<br>Narrated PowerPoint presentation<br>Podcasts<br>Reading<br>Pre-course assessment | Educator | 1–2 months pre-session |
| Book & confirm venue | Administrator | 2 months pre-session |
| Book & confirm faculty | Administrator | 2 months pre-session |
| Advertise and invite learners | Administrator | 2 months pre-session |
| Communicate with faculty | Administrator & Educator | 1 month pre-session |
| Communicate with learners | Administrator | 1 month pre-session |
| Draw up equipment list | Educator & Tech | 2 months pre-session |
| Book equipment and order consumables | Tech & Administrator | 2–3 months pre-session |
| Confirm tech required | Educator & Tech | 2–3 months pre-session |
| Develop session evaluation form | Educator | 1–2 months pre-session |
| Distribute session evaluations | Administrator | On day of session |
| Collate session evaluations | Administrator | Within 1 week of session |
| Feedback course evaluation to faculty | Administrator | Within 1 week of session |

## Learners

Preparing learners for a skills session may involve sending out learning materials in advance. This can facilitate in-depth discussion during the session and enables further engagement and active learning of the learners; it also facilitates discussion of new concepts in a more informed manner as a consequence of pre-reading, saving time on the day (Gilboy et al., 2015). The content should be relevant and succinct to ensure that the learners engage and complete the materials ahead of time (Gilboy et al., 2015; MacManaway, 1970).

When planning a practical skills session, there are things to consider. To help guide the educator, the following questions should be answered at the outset:

1. Who is the learner group?
2. Which skill are you planning to teach?
3. Why is it necessary for them to learn this skill?
4. Is this a new skill, or does it build on a previous skill, e.g., peripheral venous cannulation after learning venepuncture?
5. Is pre-learning required, and how will this be delivered – book, podcast, video?
6. Who should teach this skill, and do they have clinical credibility?
7. How will this skill be evaluated?
8. Who should evaluate?
9. What are the criteria for satisfactory completion?

The answers to these questions will be determined by the facilitator in the context of the skill session being delivered.

## The Skills Session

Like any other facilitated learning experience, a skills session must be planned in advance. Whilst planning has been considered previously in a more general context, it is also necessary to consider the production of a lesson plan, for which there are various methods, e.g., Table 5.3. However, in terms of structuring the session to promote deep learning, which will transfer to practice, Gagne's (1985) nine steps of instructional design is commonly used as part of mastery learning. This nine-step approach also transfers readily to teaching skills in health and care. Table 5.4 aligns these steps to a clinical skills session. It is important to create a positive and constructive learning environment, where learners feel it is safe to make mistakes. Should learners feel uncomfortable, vulnerable, or distracted, they will not engage effectively with the session, nor will they be able to give your carefully planned session their full attention.

| TABLE 5.3 | | | |
|---|---|---|---|
| **Lesson Plan** | | | |
| **Title** | **Date** | **Duration** | **Venue** |
| ABG Workshop | | 150 minutes | Clinical skills teaching area |
| **Level** | **Number of Learners** | | **Facilitators** |
| 4th year medical students | 8 | | 2 |
| ***Aim*** | | | |
| ■ To provide medical students with the opportunity, through facilitated workshops, to understand their critical role in the safe taking of ABGs and interpretation of results. | | | |
| ***Learning Outcomes (using Bloom's taxonomy)*** | | | |
| ■ By the end of the session students will be able to:<br>  ■ Recognise the indications for an ABG (**knowledge**)<br>  ■ Identify the landmarks to carry out an ABG (**understand**)<br>  ■ Summarise the contraindications and the complications of an ABG (**understand**)<br>  ■ Establish how to consent a patient about to undergo an ABG (**apply**)<br>  ■ Demonstrate safe acquisition of arterial blood (**apply**)<br>  ■ Interpret and analyse the results of the ABG (**analyse**)<br>  ■ Evaluate the technique of your peers through feedback (**evaluate**) | | | |

*Continued*

### TABLE 5.3 (Continued)
### Lesson Plan

**Equipment (environment):**

- Laptop & smart board
- PowerPoint presentations of:
  - Indications, contraindications and complications, arterial blood supply and anatomy
  - Modified Allen's test, landmarks to look out for
  - Pictures of ABG equipment used in local clinical practice areas
- Six case studies to discuss interpretation of results using step wise approach to ABGs
- Chairs for students and tutor

**Equipment (for skill):**

- Two manikins (high fidelity)
- Two task trainer blood gas arms to replace the manikin's normal arm and sit on the bed as though it belongs to manikin
- Beds or trolleys for 'patients' to lie in
- Personal protective equipment (PPE): Aprons, gloves, ± visors
- ABG syringes
- Sterile alcohol wipes
- Sharps disposal bin
- Swabs

| Session | Time | Activity | Resources | Other Information |
|---------|------|----------|-----------|-------------------|
| 1 | 15 mins | Introductions, aim & learning outcomes, and format of the session | PowerPoint Smart board/flipchart | Explain they might want to download the local policy and guidelines app. |
| 2 | 30 mins | Review pre-course learning material and explore experiences of practice | Facilitator's guide of pre-course material with answers | Engagement in pre-course material is a pre-requisite for attending. |
| 3 | 75 mins | Demonstration and practice of the skill | PPE Disposal bags ABG equipment Part task trainer With artificial arterial blood Skills checklists | Opportunity to practice the technique, observed by peers who will use skill checklist and provide feedback on performance. |
| 4 | 60 mins | ABG case studies | PowerPoint | After presenting 5-steps approach, allow to work in pairs to review results and their diagnosis before taking learners through the stages. |
| 5 | 15 mins | Reflection and feedback | Smart board/flipchart | Encourage reflection of the session. |
| 6 | 30 mins | Closing session Review learning outcomes | Smart board/projector/PC or laptop Participant response system/flipchart | Time for post session interactive quiz. Allow for any final questions and take home messages for future practice. Signpost for further reading/consolidation of practice. Ask learners to complete post-session evaluation. Signpost learner to post-session online questionnaire and information on OSCE. |

| Session | Facilitator Notes | | | |
|---------|-------------------|--|--|--|
| 1 | Introduce yourself and allow learners to introduce themselves. Explore learners' personal learning objectives for the session. Overview of housekeeping and session breaks. | | | |
| 2 | Allow time to explore their experience of ABG sampling, operating gas analyser and interpretation of results. | | | |

| | TABLE 5.3 (Continued) |
|---|---|
| | **Lesson Plan** |
| Session | Facilitator Notes |
| 3 | How to undertake procedure using PPE and role-modelling real practice. |
| | Emphasise the importance of explaining the procedure to gain patient cooperation and consent and role model this. |
| | Provide instructional support as needed (include discussion of type I vs type II respiratory failure, acidosis and the conditions that may give rise to abnormalities on ABG results), during the practical component after peer feedback. |
| | Adopt varied learning strategies to accommodate different learning styles: discussion, PowerPoint, peer feedback, role playing (gaining consent from me), visualising real-life practice and case examples and give examples from your own experience to emphasise learning points. |
| | Present potential complications of procedure and strategies to avoid these. Provide demonstration of technique involved in modified Allen's test to ensure collateral blood supply in event of blood clot formation after test and prevent catastrophic tissue death of hand. |
| 4 | Use PowerPoint to present cases of unwell patients needing ABGs, then in case-based discussion as required. |
| | Introduce Resuscitation Council (UK) 5 steps to ABG analysis: |
| | Step 1 – how is the patient? |
| | Step 2 – is the patient hypoxaemic? |
| | Step 3 – is the patient acidaemic or alkalaemic? |
| | Step 4 – what happened to the $PaCO_2$? |
| | Step 5 – what has happened to the base excess (BE) or bicarbonate? |
| | Discussion re expected results and why they predict that will be case. |
| | Provide real-life ABG printouts. |
| 5 | A great opportunity to highlight the benefits of reflection and reflective practice. |
| 6 | Use participant response system for end of session quiz. Allow for any final questions and take home messages for future practice. This is a good opportunity to signpost learners to any for further reading and strategies to consolidate their practice. Remember to ask learners to complete evaluation to inform future courses. |
| | Signpost learner to post-session online questionnaire and information on OSCE. |

*ABG,* Arterial blood gas; *OSCE,* Objective Structured Clinical Examination.

## *Time Out*

Using the lesson plan as an example, now begin to plan your session. Complete the sections below and write two ILOs for your session which align to Bloom's taxonomy (do not forget the verbs).

| Title | Date | Duration | Venue |
|---|---|---|---|
| | | | |

| Level | Number of Learners | Facilitators |
|---|---|---|
| | | |

| Aim |
|---|
| |

| Learning Outcomes (using Bloom's taxonomy) |
|---|
| |

| Equipment (environment): |
|---|
| |

| Equipment (for skill): |
|---|
| |

## BRIEFING

Every simulation learning environment should be a safe space for the learner. By agreeing ground rules with learners and determining the expectations of both the learners and facilitator, a learning partnership can be developed. It is also a good idea to explore with learners any previous experience of the skill about to be undertaken. This will promote learner engagement and address any ambiguity relating to the skill.

The briefing section of the session aligns with steps one to three of Gagne's nine-step structure (Gagne, 1985). As with all simulation activities, the briefing session should set the scene for the learner. It should include a review of the ILOs of the sessions and the expected learning outcomes following a period of consolidation. It is important to remember that ILOs are statements of the knowledge or skills that a learner can expect to acquire, understand, or express after completing a teaching session (Kennedy, 2006). They should therefore ideally be formed using Blooms' taxonomy of learning (1956) (Fig. 5.2). This will guide learners gradually through more sophisticated levels of thinking, starting with knowledge and comprehension levels at the base level, moving through to analysis and eventually evaluation levels of thinking.

To allow the learner to get the most from the skills session, the briefing session should be used to familiarise learners with the equipment and manikins or training models that will be used. This is a good opportunity to inform the learners of the functionality of these, and what they can and cannot do.

When a flipped classroom approach has been used, the briefing session should allow time for learners to ask questions relating to pre-session material. This will enable clarification of any points they are unsure of. This also provides an opportunity for facilitators to reinforce the most recent evidence base for the skill.

### Time Out

Using Table 5.5 as a guide, where we present an example of the application of Gagne's structure to planning, delivering, and evaluating a practical skills session, complete the template for the briefing stage of your skills session.

| TABLE 5.4 | | |
|---|---|---|
| **Steps 1–3 of Gagne's Events of Instruction** | | |
| **Gagne's Events of Instruction** | **Activity to Produce Event** | **Examples Used in Your Skills Session** |
| 1. Gain attention | Opening activity to set the scene and engage learners. | |
| 2. Inform learners of objectives | Present intended learning objectives using Bloom's taxonomy. | |
| 3. Stimulate recall of prior learning | Facilitate discussion of pre-course learning. | |

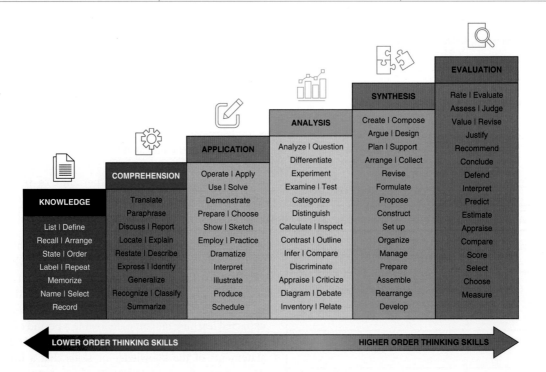

**Fig. 5.2** ■ Bloom's taxonomy verb chart. (Data from https://tips.uark.edu/blooms-taxonomy-verb-chart/ Posted by Jessica Shabatura. Sep 18 2014.)

| | TABLE 5.5 | | |
|---|---|---|---|
| | **Application of Gagne's Events of Instruction** | | |
| | **Gagne's Events of Instruction** | **Activity to Produce Event** | **Examples Used in Skills Session** |
| Briefing | 1. Gain attention | Opening activity to set the scene and engage learners. | ▪ Ask any previous experience or practice in real patients or skills labs<br>▪ Ask any previous experience interpreting results – what was the context?<br>▪ Explain competency required by professional body<br>▪ Explain this is a painful and potentially dangerous procedure for patients to undergo and therefore necessary to cover<br>▪ Ask learners what they want to achieve from session (personal objectives) |
| | 2. Inform learners of objectives | Present intended learning objectives using Bloom's taxonomy. | By the end of the session learners will be able to:<br>▪ Recognise the indications for an arterial blood gas (ABG) (understand)<br>▪ Identify the landmarks to carry out an ABG (understand)<br>▪ Summarise the contraindications and the complications of an ABG (understand)<br>▪ Establish how to consent a patient about to undergo an ABG (apply)<br>▪ Demonstrate safe acquisition of arterial blood (apply)<br>▪ Interpret and analyse the results of the ABG (analyse)<br>▪ Evaluate the technique of your peers through feedback (evaluate) |
| | 3. Stimulate recall of prior learning | Facilitate discussion of pre-course learning. | Review pre-course learning material and explore experiences of practice. Consider:<br>▪ Have learners seen an ABG done?<br>▪ Have they interpreted gases before?<br>▪ What did the printout look like?<br>▪ What were they looking for?<br>▪ Did the results mean anything? |
| Delivery | 4. Presenting stimulant materials | Delivery of new content in small chunks of time (e.g., 10–15 min intervals). Relate to clinical experience, use memory prompts. | ▪ Introduce learners to the equipment and its safe use<br>▪ Demonstration of modified Allen's test<br>▪ Demonstration of ABG on low-fidelity task trainer attached to high-fidelity manikin |
| | 5. Learning guidance and guiding the student | Varied learning strategies – discussion, PowerPoint, peer feedback, role playing (gaining consent), practice. | ▪ Gaining patient consent<br>▪ Undertaking procedure using personal protective equipment<br>▪ Provide instructional support as needed in initial discussion to include type I vs type II respiratory failure, acidosis and the conditions that may give rise to abnormalities on ABG results<br>▪ Demonstration of technique involved in modified Allen's test |

*Continued*

| | TABLE 5.5 (Continued) | | |
|---|---|---|---|
| | **Application of Gagne's Events of Instruction** | | |
| | **Gagne's Events of Instruction** | **Activity to Produce Event** | **Examples Used in Skills Session** |
| | 6. Elicit performance | Allow time to practice. | ■ Role-modelling real practice<br>■ Practice on ABG part task trainer<br>■ Use Peyton's four-stage approach:<br>  ■ Demonstration of ABG on low-fidelity task trainer<br>  ■ Demonstrate with dialogue<br>  ■ Demonstrate with learner commentary<br>  ■ Demonstration by the learner<br>■ PowerPoint of cases of unwell patients needing ABGs<br>■ Discussion re expected results and why they predict that will be case |
| | 7. Provide feedback | Provide immediate, specific, and corrective feedback. | ■ Learners encourage to ask questions during practice<br>■ Learner feedback from both peers (using checklist) and instructors by group discussions<br>■ Unsafe practice recognised and corrected |
| | 8. Evaluating what has been learned | Assess learning throughout the sessions and post-course. | ■ Application of skill to case studies, which allowed learners and facilitators to assess knowledge and understanding<br>■ End of session interactive quiz |
| Debriefing | 9. Ensuring the permanence and transfer of what has been learned | Provides resources to enhance retention and facilitate transfer of knowledge. | ■ Assess performance against all of the learning outcomes<br>■ Summarise and get learners to give take-home messages<br>■ End of session interactive quiz<br>■ Visualising real-life practice, and problem solving<br>■ Provide case examples of real life ABG printouts<br>■ Post-session online questionnaire<br>■ OSCE |

## DELIVERY

The delivery phase of teaching the skill aligns with steps four to eight of Gagne's structure. When delivering practical teaching sessions, facilitators should consider the ideal way in which to teach a practical skill. One example is an approach advocated by the National Resuscitation Councils, internationally, to teach technical skills through an adaptation of Peyton's model (Bullock, 2000; Nikendei et al., 2014). This model is a systematic approach to instruction where the learner develops an understanding of the skill through observation, listening and finally practice. Nikendei et al. (2014) described this as:

- Step one: Demonstration
  The practical skill is performed by an instructor in real time without commentary (to allow the learner to see what is expected of them by the end of the session).
- Step two: Deconstruction
  The facilitator repeats the performance of the practical skill, in the same order as step one,

this time with additional vocal commentary to explain the procedure.
- Step three: Comprehension
  The facilitator performs the practical skill, again in the same order, this time inviting a learner to commentate on the steps they see.
- Step four: Performance
Real time practice of the skill by the learner with their own spoken commentary, along with feedback and correction from the facilitator.

The benefit of a standardised delivery of teaching using Peyton's model is twofold: all learners develop the same skills in the same manner, facilitating quality assurance in the teaching process in a reproducible method. The other value is that of greater team cohesion because there is an understanding of roles and responsibilities. Using Peyton's four-step approach to teach in a skills laboratory setting has been shown to be superior in developing professionalism, communication, and skills competence of learners (Nikendei et al.,

2014). Additionally, it has been found that this approach reduces the time taken for novices to acquire new techniques when compared to standard bedside teaching methods (Krautter et al., 2011; Lund et al., 2012).

Thought should be given to the strategy for evaluating learning throughout the session. Validated tools may be useful for this purpose such as global rating scales, or a peer checklist comprising of the individual components of the skill (see section on Mastery-Based Learning, earlier) (Table 5.6). Learners should not feel rushed when honing skills in a learning environment and time should be allowed for questions and reflection in-action (as they perform the skill), after which the session should be closed appropriately and in a timely way

### Time Out

Using the completed Table 5.5 as an exemplar, complete the template (Table 5.7) for the delivery component of your skill teaching session. This aligns to steps four to eight of Gagne's structure (Gagne, 1985) and teaching the skill itself may include an adaptation of Peyton's model in stage 4.

## DEBRIEFING

Feedback is an essential element of a skills session: time should be dedicated throughout, and at the end of the session, to enable learners to reflect, discuss, and describe their experience. Aspects of this align to steps eight and nine of Gagne's event of instruction (see Table 5.5). As a facilitator of learning, your role is to guide discussion and feedback. Advocacy with enquiry is one style of feedback (Hardavella et al., 2017) which allows learners to consider their practical experience when engaging in discussion with the facilitator, subject matter expert, or peer, and this forms the basis of experiential learning (Carpendale and Ulrich, 2004; Dewey, 1933, 1938; Kaufmann and Mann, 2014; Lewin, 1951). The facilitation of the reflection process should be led by the learners, and their active participation encouraged by the teaching faculty.

### Debriefing and Learning Through Reflection

The most common reflective model which is applied in modern health and care education was set out by Kolb in 1984. Kolb (1984) suggests learning is a process based on

experience, and that this occurs through a series of four interlinked stages in a continuous learning cycle (Fig. 5. 3) (Friedman et al., 2002; Kolb, 1984; Vince, 1998). When learners repeatedly progress around the cycle, actively experimenting and reflecting, the complexity of tasks that learners can manage increases, and the cycle subsequently becomes a spiral of learning (Friedman et al., 2002; Kolb, 1984). The learner transforms as they climb this spiral and the most critical part of this transformation occurs through reflection, which drives adult learning (Kolb and Fry, 1975; Nestel and Tierney, 2007) and continuous professional development (Girvan et al., 2016; Kaufmann and Mann, 2014; Kolb and Kolb, 2006; Minott, 2010). This is fundamental to all health and care professionals where life-long learning and reflection are essential for personal growth and professional practice.

Learning in simulated practice will be enhanced when reflection on action (after the event) occurs (Ker and Bradley, 2014; Kolb, 1984; Lederman, 1992; Motola et al., 2013). Without facilitated reflection on the simulation experience, there may be missed opportunities for correcting errors. Peer-review is a strategy which enables reflective and collaborative learning.

### How to Facilitate the Debrief Session

This should begin with a learning conversation, where the facilitator capitalises on the trust developed throughout the session to stimulate open and transparent communication with the learners. The facilitator's role is to guide the learner by listening to their interpretation and reflection on events, to generate discussion, offer constructive feedback, and ultimately link this to the predetermined ILOs. This is also referred to as 'closing the loop' in the communication. Examples of questions which could guide the debriefing component of the session include:

- Tell me what worked well.
- What did you find challenging?
- What in particular was challenging about the skill?
- What would you like to review again?
- How will you apply what you have done today in your clinical setting?

In situations where audio-visual technology is available, and the skill has been recorded, it may be worth spending time to review this to highlight learning points, particularly in relation to examples of good practice. Earlier in the chapter we discussed the use

## TABLE 5.6

### Arterial Blood Gas Peer Checklist

| Preparation | Achieved |
|---|---|
| Gathers equipment with minimal assistance:<br>■ Personal protective equipment (PPE)<br>■ Skin cleanser<br>■ Arterial blood gas (ABG) syringe<br>■ Dry swabs<br>■ Sharps disposal | |
| Introduces self & confirms patient identity | |
| Explains the procedure to check there are no contraindications and gain consent | |
| Undertakes modified Allen's test<br>■ Asks patient to make closed fist, occlude both radial and ulnar arteries; patient opens palm which should be pale; release ulnar artery and then time duration for palm reperfusions (normal <5s); repeat for radial artery. | |

| Procedure | Achieved |
|---|---|
| Performs hand hygiene | |
| Puts on appropriate size of gloves | |
| Positions patient's wrist | |
| Cleanses area with skin cleanser | |
| Offers local anaesthetic, checking for allergies | |
| Checks if ABG syringe requires air to be expelled and does this | |
| Re-palpates radial artery with non-dominant index and middle finger, proximal to point of intended needle insertion | |
| Inserts ABG needle and syringe at 30–45 degree angle, immediately below fingers into the point of pulsation | |
| Awaits flashback of blood into ABG syringe | |
| Holds syringe still, does not pull back on plunger | |
| Achieves adequate sample of at least 1 mL | |
| Withdraws needle steadily and immediately applies pressure to puncture site using non-sterile gauze | |

| Post-Procedure | |
|---|---|
| Ensures pressure applied to the area for minimum 3 mins | |
| Removes needle from syringe and expels air | |
| Applies cap to end of syringe | |
| Safely disposes of sharps in sharps box | |
| Gently inverts syringe to ensure heparin mixed through | |
| Labels sample with patient's details | |
| Prepares to send sample for analysis in correct receptacle | |
| Arranges for analysis, documenting $FiO_2$ & temperature | |
| Documents procedure | |

| General Considerations | |
|---|---|
| Maintained communication with patient | |
| Smooth transition between procedural steps | |
| Aseptic non-touch technique maintained throughout | |

TABLE 5.7

**Template for Delivery**

| Gagne's Event of Instruction (Steps 4–8) | Activity to Produce Event | Examples Used in Skills Session |
|---|---|---|
| 4. Presenting stimulant materials | Delivery of new content in small chunks of time (e.g., 10–15 min intervals). Relate to clinical experience, use memory prompts. | |
| 5. Learning guidance and guiding the student | Varied learning strategies – discussion, PowerPoint, peer feedback, role playing (gaining consent), practice. | |
| 6. Elicit performance | Allow time to practice. | |
| 7. Provide feedback | Provide immediate, specific, and corrective feedback. | |
| 8. Evaluating what has been learned | Assess learning throughout the sessions and post-course. | |

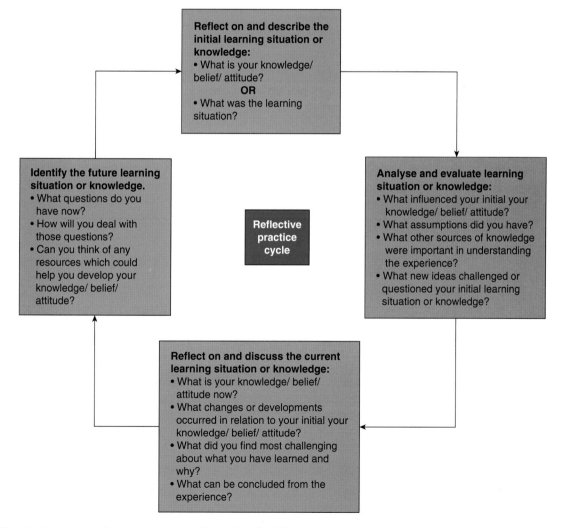

Fig. 5.3 ■ Adapted reflective practice cycle (From Kolb, D. 1984. Experiential learning: Experience as the source of learning and development. Englewood Cliffs, N.J.; London: Prentice Hall; Gibbs, G. 1988. Learning by doing: A guide to teaching and learning methods. Further Education Unit. Oxford: Oxford Polytechnic; Wight, I., Kellett, J., Pieters, J., 2016. Practice~ reflection~ learning: Work experience in planner education. Plan Pract Res, 31(5), 500-512.)

of a skills procedure checklist as an aide memoir for learners as a peer assessment tool. This ensures best practice, as there will be standardisation of the skill being taught and this provides quality assurance.

Based on step nine of Gagne's structure, strategies can be put in place to measure the transfer of learning to practice, for example, follow up online questionnaires, or practical examinations in the form of OSCEs (Objective Structured Clinical Examinations). When assessing skills acquisition, this must be gauged according to both the level of the learner and whether or not the ILOs have been met.

### Time Out

Using Table 5.7 as an exemplar, complete the template for your planned skill session.

| 8. Evaluating what has been learned | Assess learning throughout the sessions and post-course. | |
|---|---|---|
| 9. Ensuring the permanence and transfer of what has been learned | Provides resources to enhance retention and facilitate transfer of knowledge. | |

## TOP TIPS

The following are some top tips to consider on your journey to developing and delivering a simulation-based skills session.

| Top Tip | Guidance |
|---|---|
| ▪ Location, location, location | Try to find a location for your session which has the balance of being located conveniently for learners, but preferably not immediately next to a clinical area. Good lighting and handwashing facilities are important features. |

| Top Tip | Guidance |
|---|---|
| ▪ It's not only make-believe! Creating an authentic experience | Use a checklist you can add to, or refer to, prior to each session. Run through the procedure or scenario and outline the equipment you will need at each stage. It is important to access equipment used within normal patient settings to allow for realism to be integral to any skills and procedures being taught. |
| ▪ Teamwork makes a dream work | It is important to remember all members of the simulation faculty contribute to the learner's experience. Value the contribution of all faculty members and include them from the outset. Everyone may have specific skills but by bringing these together, you will become a finely choreographed simulation team who will provide an excellent learner experience. |
| ▪ It's all in the planning | Plan your session ahead of time and use a lesson plan structure. A good lesson plan should allow for some degree of flexibility, as without this, you may experience unnecessary stress trying to cram in detail. |
| ▪ Maintain a safe learning environment throughout | When using audio-visual for feedback in the debrief, it may be tempting to use examples of mistakes or errors as a teaching point. Please do not do this! The learner will remember the negative feelings more than the positives, and this does not foster a safe learning environment. |

## SUMMARY

This chapter has explored the various ways to teach practical skills in a simulation environment. It should now be clear, as part of this exploration, that each approach presents both challenges and opportunities. Irrespective of these, the development of contextual knowledge and understanding should assist the reader to develop the confidence required to plan and develop an educationally robust simulated skills session, underpinned by relevant education theory. Whilst the session may not be perfect at first attempt, engaging in reflection with the simulation faculty, as well as reviewing learners' evaluations of the session, will enable you to gain valuable insight regarding any changes required to enhance future delivery of the session.

## REFERENCES

Bandura, A., 1986. Social Foundations of Thought and Action. A Social Cognitive Theory. Prentice-Hall, Englewood Cliffs, NJ.

Bloom, B., 1956. Taxonomy of Educational Objectives: The Classification of Educational Goals. Longmans, Green, New York.

Bullock, I., 2000. Skill acquisition in resuscitation. Resuscitation 45 (2), 139–143.

Burford, B., Whittle, V., Vance, G.H., 2014. The relationship between medical student learning opportunities and preparedness for practice: a questionnaire study. BMC Medical Education 14 (1), 1–8.

Carpendale, J., Ulrich, M., 2004. Social Interaction and the Development of Knowledge. Lawrence Erlbaum Associates, Mahwah, NJ. Chapter 3.

Chamberland, M., Mamede, S., St-Onge, C., Setrakian, J., Bergeron, L., Schmidt, H., 2015. Self-explanation in learning clinical reasoning: the added value of examples and prompts. Medical Education 49 (2), 193–202.

Croskerry, P., 2009. Clinical cognition and diagnostic error: applications of a dual process model of reasoning. Advances in Health Science Education (14), 27–35. https://doi.org/10.1007/s10459-009-9182-2.

Dewey, J., 1933. How We Think. D.C. Heath & CO Publishers, Boston.

Dewey, J., 1938. Experience and Education. Kappa Delta Phi, Touchstone, New York, NY.

Dreyfus, S.E., Dreyfus, H.L., 1980. A Five-Stage Model of the Mental Activities Involved in Directed Skill Acquisition. California University Berkeley Operations Research Center, Berkeley, California.

Egan, T., Jaye, C., 2009. Communities of clinical practice: the social organization of clinical learning. Health 13 (1), 107–125.

Ericsson, K., 2004. Deliberate practice and the acquisition and maintenance of expert performance in medicine and related domains. Academic Medicine 79 (suppl), S70–81.

Ericsson K: An expert-performance perspective of research on medical expertise: the study of clinical performance, Medical Education 41:1124–1130, 2007.

Ericsson, K.A., Krampe, R.T., Tesch-Römer, C., 1993. The role of deliberate practice in the acquisition of expert performance. Psychological Review 100 (3), 363.

Ericsson K, Lehmann A: Expert and exceptional performance: evidence of maximal adaptation to task constraints, Annual Review of Psychology 47(1):273–305, 1996, https://doi.org/10.1146/annurev.psych.47.1.273.

Friedman, A., Watts, D., Croston, J., Durkin, C., 2002. Evaluating online cpd using educational criteria derived from the experiential learning cycle. British Journal of Educational Technology 33 (4), 367–378.

Gagne, R., 1985. The Conditions of Learning and Theory of Instruction Robert Gagné. Holt, Rinehart & Winston, New York, NY.

General Medical Council, 2018. Outcomes for Graduates 2018. [online] Available at https://www.gmc-uk.org/-/media/documents/practical-skills-and-procedures-a4_pdf-78058950. Accessed 31st December 2022.

Gibbs, G., 1988. Learning by Doing: A Guide to Teaching and Learning Methods. Further Education Unit. Oxford Polytechnic, Oxford.

Gilboy, M.B., Heinerichs, S., Pazzaglia, G., 2015. Enhancing student engagement using the flipped classroom. Journal of Nutrition Education and Behavior 47 (1), 109–114.

Girvan C, Conneely C, Tangney B: Extending experiential learning in teacher professional development, teaching and teacher education 58:129–139, 2016.

Health Care Professions Council, 2022. Standards of Proficiency [online] Available at https://www.hcpc-uk.org/standards/standards-of-proficiency/reviewing-the-standards-of-proficiency/. Accessed 31st December 2022.

Hardavella, G., Aamli-Gaagnat, A., Saad, N., Rousalova, I., Sreter, K.B., 2017. How to give and receive feedback effectively. Breathe 13 (4), 327–333.

Higgs, J., Jones, M., 2008. Clinical Decision Making and Multiple Problem Spaces. In: Higgs, J., Jones, M., Loftus, S., Christensen, N. (Eds.), Clinical reasoning in the health professions, 3rd Ed. Butterworth-Heinemann, Oxford, pp. 3–18.

Illing, J.C., Morrow, G.M., Rothwell nee Kergon, C.R., Burford, B.C., Baldauf, B.K., Davies, C.L., et al., 2013. Perceptions of UK medical graduates' preparedness for practice: a multi-centre qualitative study reflecting the importance of learning on the job. BMC Medical Education 13 (1), 1–12.

Issenberg, S.B., McGaghie, W.C., Gordon, D.L., Symes, S., Petrusa, E.R., Hart, I.R., et al., 2002. Effectiveness of a cardiology review course for internal medicine residents using simulation technology and deliberate practice. Teaching and Learning in Medicine 14 (4), 223–228.

Issenberg, S.B., McGaghie, W.C., Petrusa, E.R., Lee Gordon, D., Scalese, R.J., 2005. Features and uses of high-fidelity medical simulations that lead to effective learning: a beme systematic review. Medical Teacher 27 (1), 10–28.

Joint Royal College of Physicians Training Board, 2019. Curriculum for Internal Medicine, Stage 1 Training. [online] Available at: https://www.jrcptb.org.uk/sites/default/files/Internal%20 Medicine%20stage%201%20curriculum%20FINAL%20111217. pdf. Accessed 31 December 2022.

Kauffman D, Mann K: *Teaching and learning in medical education: how theory can inform practice – in understanding medical education*. In Swanwick Tim, editor: 2nd ed., John Wiley & Sons, Ltd, 2014, (Chapter 2.

Kennedy, D., 2006. Writing and Using Learning Outcomes: A Practical Guide. University College Cork, Cork, Ireland.

Ker J, Bradley P: *Simulation in medical education, in understanding medical education: evidence, theory and practice*. In Swanwick Tim, editor: 2nd edition, The Association for the Study of Medical Education, 2014, pp 175–192, (Chapter 13.

Kim, J., Park, J.H., Shin, S., 2016. Effectiveness of simulation-based nursing education depending on fidelity: a meta-analysis. BMC Medical Education 16 (1), 1–8.

Kolb, D., 1984. Experiential Learning: Experience as the Source of Learning and Development. Prentice Hall, Englewood Cliffs, NJ. London.

Kolb, D., Fry, R., 1975. Toward an Applied Theory of Experiential Learning. In: Cooper, C. (Ed.), Theories of group process. John Wiley, London.

Kolb, A.Y., Kolb, D.A., 2006. Learning Styles and Learning Spaces: A Review of Interdisciplinary Application of Experiential Learning in Higher Education. In: Sims, R., Sims, S. (Eds.), Learning styles and learning: A key to meeting the accountability demands in education. Nova, Hauppauge, NY.

Kotsis, S.V., Chung, K.C., 2013. Application of see one, do one, teach one concept in surgical training. Plastic and Reconstructive Surgery 131 (5), 1194.

Krautter, M., Weyrich, P., Schultz, J.H., Buss, S.J., Maatouk, I., Jünger, J., et al., 2011. Effects of Peyton's four-step approach on objective performance measures in technical skills training: a controlled trial. Teaching and Learning in Medicine 23 (3), 244–250.

Krautter M, Dittrich R, Safi A, Krautter J, Maatouk I, Moeltner A, Herzog W, Nikendei C: Peyton's four-step approach: differential effects of single instructional steps on procedural and memory performance – a clarification study, *Advances in Medical Education and Practice* 6:399–406, 2015, https://doi.org/10.2147/AMEP.S81923.

Lave, J., Wenger, E., 1991. Situated Learning: Legitimate Peripheral Participation. Cambridge University Press, Cambridge.

Lederman, L.C., 1992. Debriefing: toward a systematic assessment of theory and practice. Simulation & Gaming 23 (2), 145–160.

Lewin, K., 1951. Field Theory in Social Sciences. Harper & Row, New York, NY.

Lund, F., Schultz, J.H., Maatouk, I., Krautter, M., Möltner, A., Werner, A., et al., 2012. Effectiveness of IV cannulation skills laboratory training and its transfer into clinical practice: a randomized, controlled trial. PloS One 7 (3), e32831.

MacManaway, L., 1970. Teaching methods in higher education—innovation and research. Higher Education Quarterly 24, 321–329.

Mann, K., 2011. Theoretical perspectives in medical education: past experience and future possibilities. Medical Education 45 (1), 60–68.

Maran, N.J., Glavin, R.J., 2003. Low-to high-fidelity simulation–a continuum of medical education? Medical Education 37, 22–28.

McGaghie, W.C., Barsuk, J.H., Wayne, D.B. (Eds.), 2020. Comprehensive Healthcare Simulation: Mastery Learning in Health Professions Education. Springer Nature, Berlin.

McGuire, C., Hurley, R.E., Babbott, D., Butterworth, J.S., 1964. Auscultatory skill: gain and retention after intensive instruction. Academic Medicine 39 (2), 120–131.

Minott, M.A., 2010. Reflective teaching as self–directed professional development: building practical or work–related knowledge. Professional Development in Education 36 (1-2), 325–338.

Monrouxe, L.V., Bullock, A., Gormley, G., Kaufhold, K., Kelly, N., Roberts, C.E., et al., 2018. New graduate doctors' preparedness for practice: a multistakeholder, multicentre narrative study. BMJ Open 8 (8), e023146.

Motola, I., Devine, L., Chung, H., Sullivan, J., Issenberg, B., 2013. Simulation in healthcare education: a best evidence practical guide. AMEE Guide No. 82. Medical Teacher 35 (10), e1511–e1530. https://doi.org/10.3109/0142159X.2013.818632.

Murphy, J.I., 2004. Using focused reflection and articulation to promote clinical reasoning: an evidence-based teaching strategy. Nursing Education Perspectives 25 (5), 226–231.

Nestel, D., Tierney, T., 2007. Role-play for medical students learning about communication: guidelines for maximising benefits. BMC Medical Education 7 (1), 1–9.

Norman, G., 2005. Research in clinical reasoning: past history and current trends. Medical Education 39 (4), 418–427.

Nikendei, C., Zeuch, A., Dieckmann, P., Roth, C., Schäfer, S., Völkl, M., et al., 2005. Role-playing for more realistic technical skills training. Medical Teacher 27 (2), 122–126.

Nikendei, C., Huber, J., Stiepak, J., Huhn, D., Lauter, J., Herzog, W., et al., 2014. Modification of Peyton's four-step approach for small group teaching–a descriptive study. BMC Medical Education 14 (1), 1–10.

Nursing and Midwifery Council, 2018. Future Nurse: Standards of Proficiency for Registered Nurses. [online] Available at https://www.nmc.org.uk/globalassets/sitedocuments/standards-of-proficiency/nurses/future-nurse-proficiencies.pdf. Accessed 31 December 2022.

O'Sullivan, Í., Jeavons, R., 2005. Survey of blood gas interpretation. Emergency Medicine Journal 22 (5), 391–392.

Peyton, J.R. (Ed.), 1998. Teaching & Learning in Medical Practice. Manticore Europe Limited, Heronsgate Rickmansworth, UK.

Vince, R., 1998. Behind and beyond Kolb's learning cycle. Journal of Management Education 22 (3), 304–319.

Simpson, H., 2004. Interpretation of arterial blood gases: a clinical guide for nurses. British Journal of Nursing 13 (9), 522–528.

Wayne, D.B., Butter, J., Siddall, V.J., Fudala, M.J., Wade, L.D., Feinglass, J., et al., 2006. Mastery learning of advanced cardiac life support skills by internal medicine residents using simulation technology and deliberate practice. Journal of General Internal Medicine 21 (3), 251–256.

Wight, I., Kellett, J., Pieters, J., 2016. Practice- reflection- learning: work experience in planner education. Planning Practice & Research 31 (5), 500–512.

Williams, K., Leong, S.A., Gill, A., 2013. A survey of arterial blood gas use and analysis in respiratory inpatients. European Respiratory Journal 42 (Suppl. 57), 3358.

Ziv, A., Ben-David, S., Ziv, M., 2005. Simulation based medical education: an opportunity to learn from errors. Medical Teacher 27 (3), 193–199.

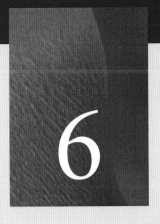

# 6

# INTERPROFESSIONAL SIMULATION

CATIE PATON ■ ELIZABETH SIMPSON ■ FIONA BURTON
■ SHARON DONAGHY ■ CAROLINE MARTIN

## CHAPTER OUTLINE

## OBJECTIVES

*This chapter should support the reader to develop an understanding of the:*

- Concept of simulation-based education (SBE) in the context of interprofessional learning (IPL).
- Background which underpins the development of SBE as part of interprofessional learning.
- Implementation of interprofessional education (IPE) as part of team learning.
- Role SBE plays in forging teams in practice, using a case study.

## KEY TERMS

**Interprofessional learning (learning with and from other professionals)**

**Interprofessional education**

**Multiprofessional (referring to the multitude of professionals within the healthcare team)**

**Healthcare teams**

**Health and care teams**

**Simulation-based education**

**Simulation environment**

**In-situ simulation**

## INTRODUCTION

The provision of a safe, effective health and care service relies on the education of the healthcare teams responsible for the delivery of the service. By embracing a culture of collaborative learning, where the diversity of a team is celebrated and valued, we can generate a cohesive workforce with patient safety at the core. This chapter will discuss simulation-based education (SBE) in the context of interprofessional learning (IPL) and will include an overview of the background to the development of SBE as part of IPL. A case study will be presented to enable consideration of the practical application of SBE from the specific perspective of IPL.

This approach will also guide the reader to consider their own practice and how learning from this chapter can be applied most effectively. Finally, Top Tips will summarise the key learning points.

## BACKGROUND

Organisations including the Centre for the Advancement of Interprofessional Education (CAIPE) have been developing and promoting the benefits of interprofessional education (IPE) since 1987. When advocating for IPE, this UK-based charity, with an international outreach, suggest that there must be a focus on how this collaborative practice can improve both patient safety and the effectiveness of care. IPE was defined by the World Health Organization (WHO) in 2010 as something that 'occurs when students from two or more professions learn about, from, and with each other to enable effective collaboration and improve health outcomes' (WHO, 2010, p. 7). It is not simply several professional groups participating in a joint simulation activity. It involves deliberate and purposeful integration focused on both learning *with* each other and learning *from* each other. While there is evidence demonstrating improved patient outcomes following IPL simulation, there remains an ongoing requirement to further strengthen the research base (Holmes and Mellanby, 2022). Within the UK, the benefits of IPL have been recognised by health and care professional regulatory bodies and IPL, often using simulation, is a core curriculum requirement for over two-thirds of professional programmes (CAIPE, 2021). Fundamentally, IPL is viewed as a method of improving the quality of patient care through increased understanding of other professionals' roles, while providing opportunities to cultivate communication, practice collaboration, and foster teamwork (Goolsarran et al., 2018).

IPL simulation has specifically been recommended by simulation organisations for some time, including the Society for Simulation in Healthcare (SSH) and the National League for Nursing (NLN) (SSH and NLN, 2013), and is a component in simulation best practice standards (International Nursing Association for Clinical Simulation and Learning (INACSL), 2016). SBE is a powerful way to provide meaningful IPL educational opportunities across all health and care disciplines,

at both undergraduate and postgraduate levels. Studies demonstrating the positive impact of IPL simulation can be found worldwide, covering a wide range of professional groups (Attoe et al., 2019; Carmela et al., 2022; Collins et al., 2021; Goulding et al., 2020; Kleib et al., 2021; Lee et al., 2020; Murray, 2021; Tallentire et al., 2022; Tilley et al., 2021). The philosophy of IPL in SBE is that of an active, experiential learning method which aims to authentically replicate the environments in which health and care teams work. This is a strength of IPL in simulation, as this approach also facilitates an appreciation of human factors, including non-technical skills (NTS). Examples of these are communication, situational awareness, and decision making in stressful and dynamic circumstances. This approach helps teams to understand behaviours and teamworking in low- and high-stress situations in a safe learning environment. It encourages teams to reflect on their strengths and consider where challenges lie and where latent errors may exist. Additionally, it is useful in developing respectful and positive attitudes towards other health and care professionals, while supporting a cohesive approach to improving patient outcomes.

### Overview of Simulation in Interprofessional Learning

Patients' needs cannot be met by a single health or care professional group. Provision and delivery of care requires a fusion of professionals, often with different perspectives of care delivery, and the contribution of other disciplines. The multidisciplinary team responsible for the delivery of care continues to evolve and is becoming increasingly more diverse and complex. The ability of health and care teams to work collaboratively is fundamental to the delivery of integrated high-quality, safe, and effective person-centred care. Yet for this to happen in a meaningful way relies on the readiness of the professionals involved to critically review both their own and other team members' practice. They must also embrace opportunities for learning from each other as this enables the development of a better understanding of profession-specific roles, contributions, and values.

The diversity of the health and care team means that each profession brings a unique set of skills, which are most effective when combined. However, historically, SBE has been directed at a single professional group (uniprofessional) which can be linked to the value each group of health and care professionals place on their individual professional identity (Charles & Koehn, 2020). Whilst adopting a uniprofessional training stance is appropriate and necessary in some situations, it can result in learning in silos, potentially generating stereotypical views of health and care colleagues' roles within the multiprofessional team. IPL simulation helps to challenge these stereotypes and has been identified as a means of enhancing the development of professional identity, not as a single profession, but as a team collaborative (Burford et al., 2020). With this in mind, IPE should be created as a deliberate, structured endeavour, with clear collaborative intended learning objectives (ILOs).

Although opportunities for IPL can be challenging to find, the benefits to both staff and patients warrants the time and effort. Logistically, it requires complex organisation which includes identification of, and proactive engagement with, key stakeholders from each professional group to ensure that IPL sessions are supported, relevant, and practically achievable. This strategy is crucial, particularly when several professions are involved (Charles and Koehn, 2020). Immersive simulation, specifically, is intended to provide an engaging, authentic experience for learners. This requires input from all professions at the outset, to ensure scenarios are designed and developed which are both authentic and applicable for all. This facilitates learning that can be achieved both individually and collaboratively and ensures that learners recognise that ILOs are directly related to their stage and learning needs. This approach will help to forge safe, effective person-centred team working and avoid the risk of interprofessional hierarchies.

## Interprofessional Learning In-Situ Simulation

Delivering IPL simulation in a dedicated learning environment has advantages and disadvantages. Learners can find the simulation learning environment challenging to fully engage with, particularly if there are significant fidelity conflicts with their usual clinical environment (see Chapters 4 and 5). One way to counteract these difficulties is to deliver the IPL simulation in-situ (e.g., in the clinical area where

the learners would normally work). Therefore, when planning the IPL simulation, it is important to decide on the optimal location to achieve the planned ILOs. Practicalities, including the size and available space for delivery of the simulation itself, space and facilities for debriefing, ability to observe the simulation remotely, and access to audio-visual (AV) systems, need to be considered.

The delivery of in-situ simulation takes place in the real-life clinical or working environment. However, it should be noted that, at all times, the safety of the real patients and staff will always take precedence over any learning event. Evidence suggests that this can lead to more natural responses and improve team working and clinical performance. This in turn results in learning which is easily applicable to learners' clinical practice (Gros et al., 2021). In-situ simulation can be an effective way to practice and plan for scenarios that are often infrequent but high risk to patient populations. From a clinical and care safety perspective, it provides a realistic experience for all team members and can lead to identification and resolution of latent threats, errors, or systems and processes (Shi et al., 2021). These include environmental, equipment related, protocols and guidelines, all of which have the potential to compromise safety. An example of this would be the use of in-situ simulation during the COVID-19 pandemic within emergency departments (Dharamsi et al., 2020). As with all IPL simulation, in-situ sessions should be planned with the learning needs of all team members in mind and delivered by adopting an interprofessional approach to maximise the benefits.

When staffing levels are low or clinical activity is high, it can be difficult to release staff for education. A benefit of in-situ simulation is that learners require to be released for a shorter period of time and remain on site. This means they can return to deliver patient care at short notice, should the clinical need arise.

In-situ IPL can be delivered on both small and large scale. For example, a deteriorating patient scenario can be delivered within a single clinical team, or the scenario could be extended to include colleagues from other departments. Large-scale IPL simulation can work across a spectrum of specialties to test care systems and processes, such as major haemorrhage. This scale of simulation can include simulating a patient's journey from the emergency department through to radiology, then theatre. This could involve administrative, porter, nursing, medical, and laboratory staff.

A strategy to support an in-situ simulation programme is the implementation of a simulation champion network. This team could work within the clinical environment as SBE ambassadors to facilitate and embed in-situ simulation in their areas. This requires motivated staff members, willing to seek out and capture opportunities as they arise, to deliver simulation sessions with their clinical team.

## PLANNING AN INTERPROFESSIONAL LEARNING SIMULATION

### Lesson Plan

As with all learning activities, the lesson plan is the first step. In previous chapters we have presented some learning theories and the concept of constructive alignment, and IPL simulation is no different. With this in mind, we need to start by deciding on the aims and objectives of the session. Our full lesson plan can be found in Table 6.1.

### Time Out

Use the template in Table 6.2 as a basis to formulate your lesson plan. Begin with your lesson aim and design your ILOs to achieve this. Remember to consider the level of the learners and select the appropriate learning verbs (see Chapter 5 and Bloom's taxonomy for more information) when developing the ILOs.

While your time frames may be different, our hope is that this template will help you.

| TABLE 6.1 |
|---|
| **Lesson Plan Example** |

| Title | Date | Duration | Venue |
|---|---|---|---|
| IPL Simulation (Evening on call) | | Full day: Each student 150 minutes | Clinical skills teaching area |

| Level | Number of Learners | Facilitators |
|---|---|---|
| Final year medical, nursing, and pharmacy students | 1 medical, 1 nurse per ward plus 1 medical and 1 pharmacy learner each rotation, and 1 pharmacy student each rotation | Coordinator × 1<br>Senior medics × 2<br>Nurses × 4<br>Hi-fidelity operators × 2 |

**Aim**

- To provide learners with the opportunity, through an immersive simulation experience, to understand their critical role within a team, in the safe prioritisation of care for a group of patients.

**Intended Learning Objectives (using Bloom's Taxonomy)**

- By the end of the session students will be able to:
  - Use a systematic ABCDE (Airway, Breathing, Circulation, Disability, Exposure) assessment when examining a patient (**apply**)
  - Demonstrate the use of clinical decision-making skills to prioritise workload (**apply**)
  - Recognise indications for escalation of patient's care to relevant colleagues (**knowledge**)
  - Demonstrate effective communication skills within an interprofessional team (**apply**)
  - Apply the SBAR (Situation, Background, Assessment, Recommendation) tool as a communication strategy (**apply**)
  - Demonstrate safe, accurate, appropriate medication prescribing and administration (**knowledge**)
  - Demonstrate safe, accurate documentation skills (**knowledge**)
  - Interpret, analyse, and appropriately respond to results of investigations (**analyse**)
  - Demonstrate effective time management skills (**apply**)
  - Demonstrate leadership skills through the safe and appropriate delegation of tasks (**apply**)
  - Demonstrate personal situational awareness and recognise own limitations (**self-awareness knowledge**)

| | | | |
|---|---|---|
| **TABLE 6.1 (Continued)** | | |
| **Lesson Plan Example** | | |

| Level | Number of Learners | Facilitators |
|---|---|---|
| | | |

**Equipment (environment):**

- Laptop & smart board, or flipchart and pens
- PowerPoint presentations of introduction and housekeeping
- Case studies with all relevant clinical documentation
- Access to electronic records and results
- Phones/pagers to communicate during simulation
- AV recording

**Clinical Equipment:**

- Simulated patients
- High-fidelity mannikins
- Moulage
- Scenario specific clinical equipment (see each individual scenario)
- Beds or trolleys for 'patients' to lie in
- PPE: Aprons, gloves, ± visors
- Appropriate clinical waste/sharps disposal bin

| Session | Time | Activity | Resources | Other Information |
|---|---|---|---|---|
| Pre-Session | | Review common medical conditions<br>Watch overview of the session | Virtual learning environment<br>Local guidelines and policies | Engagement in pre-course material is a prerequisite for attending. |
| 1 | 15 mins | Introductions, aim & learning outcomes, and format of the session | PowerPoint<br>Smart board<br>Flipchart & pens | Explain they might want to download the local policy and guidelines app. |
| 2 | 15 mins | SBAR handover from previous shift<br>Orientation to geographical layout of clinical area and contact numbers of colleagues (telephones and pagers) | SBAR handover sheet<br>Contact numbers | Allow an opportunity to ask questions.<br>Direct learners to local phones or pager system. |
| 3 | 55 mins | Immersive simulation | See equipment lists | Promote the 'safe learning environment' and that this is designed to be a valuable experience.<br>**Emphasise this is not a test,** and is a safe learning space. This about the learner's clinical decisions. |
| 4 | 30 mins | Hot debrief (uniprofessional) | Access to AV playback<br>Structured debriefing questions sheet | Use the template provided to take notes to guide the learners' discussion. If required, it is an opportunity for a short microteach and signpost learners to further reading resources. |
| | 30 mins | Interprofessional debrief | Access to AV playback<br>Structured debriefing questions sheet | Encourage participation from all disciplines and end the debrief with their 'Take home message' for practice. |

*Continued*

| TABLE 6.1 (Continued) | | | | |
|---|---|---|---|---|
| **Lesson Plan Example** | | | | |
| *Session* | *Time* | *Activity* | *Resources* | *Other Information* |
| 5 | 20 mins | Faculty debrief and reflection | | Please take notes throughout the day to inform our faculty debrief. From this we will be able to establish issues relating to equipment, staffing, learner and staff safety. |

| *Session* | *Facilitator Notes* |
|---|---|
| 1 | Introduce yourself and allow learners to introduce themselves. Explore learners' personal learning objectives for the session. Overview of housekeeping and session breaks. Make learners aware the AV recording is in use for debriefing and education purposes only. |
| 2 | Be supportive in responding to questions and encourage leaners to immerse themselves in the simulated learning experience. |
| 3 | **Layout**<br>■ There are a total of four ward areas in the simulated medical unit. The medical patients within the unit will consist of a combination of low-, medium- and high-fidelity manikins, and simulated patients (people).<br>■ **Please Note: <u>No</u> invasive procedures to be carried out on real patients.**<br><br>**Communication**<br>■ There will be a telephone in each ward, and doctor and pharmacist also have phones allocated to use as a means of communication.<br><br>**Session format**<br>■ Each immersion will last 55 minutes and there will be a nurse in each ward area, and an on-call pharmacist and medic who will cover all four wards.<br>■ It will begin with a handover for each learner with a list of remaining outstanding tasks.<br>■ The learner should be given the opportunity to prioritise these outstanding tasks.<br>■ Learners should begin in whichever order they feel is appropriate.<br>■ The on-call phone will be called with additional information relating to the changing acuity of patients as the session progresses.<br>■ Tasks, communication, and documentations should be carried out in real time.<br><br>**Simulation**<br>Please be aware this may be quite stressful for the learners. They may require time out for support and well-being. Please emphasise, this is:<br>■ A safe learning environment<br>■ An opportunity, experience, and learning space<br>■ Designed to be a valuable and productive experience<br>■ <u>**Not**</u> a test, and <u>**not**</u> an OSCE (Objective Structured Clinical Examination)<br>■ Designed to help learners gain confidence from successes & learn from mistakes<br>■ Designed to help learners recognise knowledge gaps. It can result in more questions than answers (please signpost learners to the relevant resources).<br>■ Designed to stretch you and be stressful. Stress should be productive not counterproductive, and you will aways have help available in scenarios (phone in room, senior available). |

| Session | Facilitator Notes |
|---------|-------------------|
| | **TABLE 6.1 (Continued)** |
| | **Lesson Plan Example** |
| 4 | **Individual Debrief (Uniprofessional)**<br>■ Delivered by profession-specific faculty members<br>■ Encourage reflection through advocacy with enquiry and facilitated discussion using probing questions<br>■ Offer constructive review of learner's performance<br>Please remember learners must leave 'safe for practice': any aspects of the session which give facilitator's cause for concern relating to underpinning knowledge of evidence-based practice and its application should be addressed through a short microteach session. Signpost learners to further reading resources.<br>**Interprofessional Debrief**<br>This takes place twice in the day, after the morning session and again after the afternoon session. It will be facilitated with representation from two professional groups (co-facilitation). It is designed in this way to promote equity in terms of numbers across the disciplines (by this stage, three medical, three pharmacy, and more than three nurses will have participated in the immersive simulation component). This prevents individual learners feeling a 'lone voice' and is aimed to enable free flow of discussion.<br>■ Please use the template provided to take notes to guide the learners' discussion.<br>■ Encourage participation from all disciplines.<br>■ End the interprofessional debrief by asking students for their 'Take home message'. What will they take into their practice from this experience? |
| 5 | **Faculty Debrief of the Day**<br>■ Please take notes throughout the day to inform our faculty debrief. From this we will be able to establish issues relating to equipment, staffing, learner, and staff safety.<br>■ Meta-debrief is an opportunity to review the ILOs and learning outcomes to assure the quality of the session and that learning remains constructively aligned. It is an opportunity to establish if the simulation is an authentic representation of the current clinical environment and if not, to establish the changes we need to make to address this.<br>■ For those facilitators wishing feedback on their debriefing skills, we can arrange this on an individual basis. |

## Logistics and Timelines

As with any simulation, planning is key. It is important to consider logistics which may include resources, equipment, consumables, time, and staff. It may be that you need to source equipment, which may need to be booked in advance, or order consumables for the session. You must have an understanding of local procurement processes and lead-in times for equipment to ensure this is available for your session to be delivered as planned. Having an appreciation of the time required to set up and break down for each session, in addition to the delivery time of the scenario, will allow you to organise as a team, as well as setting and meeting expectations of both learners and faculty. Checklists with timelines are useful tools and it may be worth considering using these to plan the session.

## Planning an In-Situ Interprofessional Learning Simulation

While in-situ simulation can be resource intensive for the simulation educator, there are benefits to the learner and their department. By delivering the session within the clinical area, learning becomes more accessible to the clinical team. Furthermore, this is with the reassurance that should clinical demand or pressures increase, the educators will adopt a flexible approach, and be willing to reschedule the session.

The ethos of SBE is learning in a safe environment. In-situ simulation is no exception to this; however, safety in this context must incorporate the safety of staff not involved in the simulation, learners, and real patients. Best practice would be to conduct a robust risk assessment of the clinical environment.

| TABLE 6.2 | | | |
|---|---|---|---|
| **Lesson Plan Template** | | | |

| *Title* | *Date* | *Duration* | *Venue* |
|---|---|---|---|
| | | | |

| *Level* | | *Number of Learners* | *Facilitators* |
|---|---|---|---|
| | | | |

**Aim**

This is a succinct statement of what would you like to achieve in this session.
You may find it helpful to consider some key questions, for example:

- Who are the target group?
- As the facilitator, what is the purpose of this interprofessional learning (IPL) experience?
- What will learners gain from this IPL experience?
- What is the IPL trying to achieve?

**Intended Learning Objectives (using Bloom's Taxonomy)**

Think here about what activities you would like learners to do to demonstrate they are achieving your aim.

**Equipment (environment):**



**Clinical Equipment:**

| *Session* | *Time* | *Activity* | *Resources* | *Other Information* |
|---|---|---|---|---|
| Pre-Session | | Review common medical conditions<br>Watch overview of the session (insert video link) | Virtual learning environment<br>Local guidelines and policies | Engagement in pre-course material is a prerequisite for attending |
| 1 | | | | |
| 2 | | | | |
| 3 | | | | |
| 4 | | | | |
| 5 | | | | |

| *Session* | *Facilitator Notes* |
|---|---|
| 1 | |
| 2 | |
| 3 | |
| 4 | |
| 5 | |

## Time Out

Table 6.3 is an example of a risk assessment used by NHS Lanarkshire in Scotland. Use this template as a basis to consider any associated risks with your in-situ simulation, and how these will be addressed. You may need to design your own assessment, but this may help you to get started.

You should discuss the consumables required for the simulation with the individual responsible for finance within the department in which the in-situ simulation will be taking place. To truly immerse learners in the session, using equipment that they are familiar with, and will use in real situations, is vital. However, this can prove expensive in some situations and may, if clinical equipment is used for the simulation, potentially impact on the availability of essential resources for clinical use.

For in-situ simulation it is essential to have a plan which promotes the safety of real patients and the equipment required to care for them. This might involve developing plans for replenishing stock of consumables post-simulation, along with a process

| TABLE 6.3 | | |
|---|---|---|
| **Risk Assessment for Simulation in Clinical Areas** | | |
| *Risk Assessment for Simulation in Clinical Areas* | | |
| Purpose: To ensure physical and psychological safety in a clinical simulated learning environment | | |
| Date | Hospital Site | Clinical Area |
| *Faculty/Roles* | | |
| | **Name** | **Role in simulation session** |
| Lead for simulation session | | |
| Other faculty | | |
| Technical support | | |
| Embedded professional (EP) | | |
| Lead for clinical area | | |
| *Housekeeping* | | |
| Suitable space available for simulation and debrief | | |
| Fire exits/drills | | |
| Toilets | | |
| Contact numbers of simulation team displayed | | |
| *Communication/Engagement* | | |
| Signage displayed | Yes | No |
| Nurse in charge and/or Dr in charge of clinical area happy that running simulation should not compromise patient safety | Please Sign | |
| Plan scenarios and faculty allocation/roles | Yes | No |
| Staff allocated to attend <br> ■ Who <br> ■ When | | |
| Authorising signature of department lead to use consumables | | |
| Authorising signature of department lead to use emergency equipment | | |
| Plan agreed for restocking consumables | Yes | No |
| Social media control in place for @nhsl_meded tweet | Yes | No |

*Continued*

| TABLE 6.3 (Continued) | | |
|---|---|---|
| **Risk Assessment for Simulation in Clinical Areas** | | |
| Social media control in place for hospital site tweet | Yes | No |
| *Safety* | | |
| Adequate faculty available | | |
| ▪ Technician present | Yes | No |
| ▪ Simulation-based educator team: 2 facilitators/1 EP/additional person if doing clinical emergency simulation | Yes | No |
| ▪ Additional volunteer if manikin not used | Yes | No |
| Ensure measures in place to maintain safety/'real' patient modifications required | Yes | No |
| Highlighted in hospital safety brief | Yes | No |
| Highlighted in department huddle | Yes | No |
| Plan for 'real world' event in place<br>▪ Discussed and agreed with clinical staff<br>▪ Discussed and agreed with simulation staff | Please detail | |
| If clinical emergency team call (2222) planned as part of simulation session:<br>▪ Clinical emergency team members know of potential simulated event.<br>▪ Switchboard aware of planned simulation and given contact number for faculty.<br>Name of allocated person to:<br>▪ Inform switchboard immediately prior to scenario starting.<br>▪ Inform switchboard at end.<br>▪ Meet 2222 team members on arrival to allow reprioritisation of clinical duties if needed. Encourage team to remain for debrief if possible. | | |
| *AV Governance* | | |
| Standard Operating Procedure for AV recording during in-situ simulation is adhered to throughout session. | Please Sign | |
| Cameras and microphones turned away from clinical area and recording stopped at end of simulation session. | | |
| ▪ Confirmed by lead for simulation<br>▪ Confirmed by lead for clinical area | Please Sign | |

to promptly finish the simulation and restore the clinical area ready to receive a patient should clinical pressures require this. Careful planning and role allocation of the faculty delivering the simulation beforehand promotes a seamless transition from simulation to real care environment. An example is the delivery of an IPL paediatric simulation in an Emergency Department that has limited paediatric resuscitation space and equipment. Establishing these processes when meeting with key stakeholders pre-simulation demonstrates appreciation of patients' and learners' conceptual, physical, and psychological safety (see Chapter 4).

## Planning Off-Site Interprofessional Learning Simulation

The planning involved for an IPL simulation activity away from the health or care environment (off site) involves dovetailing both the profession-specific and teamwork-associated ILOs. From a logistical perspective, consideration may need to be given to the commitments of learner groups and the supporting faculty. When IPL involves several professions, meeting the needs of each profession will require negotiation, clear communication, and coordination of timetables. Working together, you can reach a consensus to agree your ILOs and design your scenarios to achieve these.

With interprofessional simulation comes interprofessional faculty; this creates space and opportunities for collaboration, shared decision making, and capitalising on the diversity of skillsets across the team. These activities enable effective collegiate working towards a shared goal.

### Time Out

Using Tables 6. 4 and 6.5 as a guide, think about the simulation and what you may need to plan for your session. Remember to consider timelines and allocate the responsibilities to individuals within your team.

### Example of Interprofessional Learning Simulation (Evening on Call)

This example of 'evening on call' (Fig. 6.1) offered an opportunity for medical, nursing, and pharmacy students to experience their postgraduate roles and interprofessional team working. The immersive component of the simulation experience lasted for 55 minutes for each learner and, although this took place during the day, was designed to replicate, as authentically as possible, an out-of-hours, on-call shift. This was the result of a team collaboration, motivated by the work of Swann et al. (2008) who developed a teaching session designed to prepare medical students to work in a hospital environment, learning key skills including interprofessional working and prioritisation.

Hosted within a medical education training centre in Scotland, an 'evening on call' was designed to present a simulated medical unit, consisting of four medical specialties including an acute admissions unit, cardiology, respiratory, and endocrinology (McGregor et al., 2012). Each ward was staffed

| TABLE 6.4 | | |
|---|---|---|
| **Task List for Interprofessional Learning Simulation** | | |
| *To Do* | *Responsible* | *Timeframe* |
| | | |
| | | |
| | | |
| | | |
| | | |
| | | |
| | | |
| *In-situ specific* | | |
| Risk assessment | | |
| Confirm on the day | | |
| Discuss plan B | | |

| TABLE 6.5 | | |
|---|---|---|
| **Task Allocation List and Timelines** | | |
| **To Do** | **Responsible** | **Timeframe** |
| Write ILOs and lesson plan | Education team | 3 months pre-session |
| Develop pre-course materials:<br>　Narrated PowerPoint<br>　Podcasts<br>　Reading<br>　Pre-course assessment | Education team | 1–2 months pre-session |
| Book & confirm venue | Administrator | 2 months pre-session |
| Book & confirm faculty | Administrator | 2 months pre-session |
| Advertise and invite learners | Administrator | 2 months pre-session |
| Communicate with faculty | Administrator & coordinating educator | 1 month pre-session |
| Communicate with learners | Administrator | 1 month pre-session |
| Draw up equipment list | Education team & Sim technologist | 2 months pre-session |
| Book equipment and order consumables | Sim technologist team & administrator | 2–3 months pre-session |
| Confirm tech required | Education team & Sim technologist | 2–3 months pre-session |
| Develop session evaluation form | Coordinating educator | 1–2 months pre-session |
| Distribute end of session evaluations | Administrator | On day of session |
| Collate session evaluations | Administrator | Within 1 week of session |
| Feedback course evaluation to faculty | Administrator | Within 1 week of session |
| Arrange faculty debrief | Coordinating educator | Within 2 weeks of session |
| *In-situ specific* | | |
| Risk assessment | | |
| Confirm on the day | | |
| Discuss plan B | | |

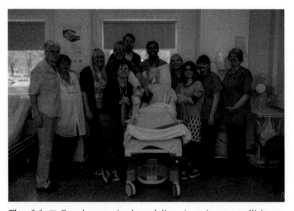

**Fig. 6.1** ■ Faculty required to deliver 'evening on call' interprofessional learning.

by one newly qualified nurse (a role undertaken by a final year nursing student) and one senior nurse (a role undertaken by a nurse educator), and all wards were covered by an on-call pharmacist. The patients across these wards consisted of a combination of low-, medium-, and high-fidelity manikins as well as simulated patients (real people).

Each medical student was allocated to the unit for their 'evening on call' to provide medical cover for all four wards. They were given a shift handover using the SBAR (Situation, Background, Assessment and Recommendation) tool (Table 6.6); this provided an overview of the patients they were responsible for, and also any outstanding tasks. Medical

**TABLE 6.6**

**Example of SBAR Handover**

| WARD | Patient Label | | PATIENTS CAUSING CONCERN/ OUTSTANDING TASKS |
|---|---|---|---|
| 1 | Elizabeth Doran<br>DOB: 04/06/1968<br>Age 53/54 | S | Diabetic ketoacidosis (DKA) admitted this morning. Confused on admission. DKA Care Pathway 2 now in progress. |
| | | B | Type 1 Diabetic, Anxiety disorder |
| | | A | Condition stabilised. Neurologically improved. Changed to DKA care pathway 2. Urinary retention – for catheter. |
| | | R | **Review re DKA care pathway, Fluids and Urea & Electrolytes (U&Es)** |
| 2 | Yvonne Graham<br>DOB: 15/07/1974<br>Age 47 | S | Admitted today with witnessed haematemesis. Condition stable. Gastro-intestinal endoscopy ordered for tomorrow am. |
| | | B | Epilepsy |
| | | A | Hgb 9.9. Stable at present. **Nil by Mouth.** |
| | | R | **Intra-venous fluids need prescribed. On call Surgeons aware of condition – please contact if any deterioration out of hours.** |
| 2 | Helen McLean<br>DOB: 18/06/1945<br>Age 76 | S | Admitted yesterday with exacerbation of chronic obstructive pulmonary disease (COPD). Type II respiratory failure. |
| | | B | COPD, Ex-smoker |
| | | A | Treated with non-invasive ventilation (NIV) now discontinued. Commenced on steroids & nebulisers. Remains dyspnoeic but condition stable on 28% $O_2$. |
| | | R | **Junior Doctor to check condition this evening.** |
| 4 | E McCluskey<br>DOB: 12/08/1969<br>Age 52 | S | Day 3 now stable following myocardial infarction (MI) and pulmonary oedema. |
| | | B | Admitted 2 days ago with anterior ST elevation myocardial infarction. Primary percutaneous coronary intervention (PPCI) carried out. Stent to left anterior descending (LAD).<br>Developed acute left ventricular failure (LVF) pulmonary oedema on day 2 @ 22.00hrs. |
| | | A | Weaned off IV diuretics and nitrates and now on oral medications. |
| | | R | **Junior Doctor to review this afternoon/evening to check no further acute LVF.** |
| 4 | Irene Stewart<br>DOB: 08/11/1944<br>Age 77 | S | Sepsis ?cause |
| | | B | Type 1 diabetes mellitus |
| | | A | Stable |
| | | R | **Gentamicin prescription required.** |
| 4 | David Smith<br>DOB: 03/12/1965<br>Age 56 | S | Admitted today with chest pain |
| | | B | Hypercholesterol, Smoker<br>GTN administered in ambulance, pain resolved. |
| | | A | 12 lead electrocardiograph (ECG) NAD. Stable since admission. Observe overnight. |
| | | R | **Troponin due @ 18.30.** |

students were asked to appropriately prioritise and manage care, and they were advised that, should they require assistance, they could ask the nurse within the ward, call a medical colleague, or contact the on-call pharmacist. Ward computers and patient records were available, helping to ensure that this simulation experience was reflective of real clinical practice (Fig. 6.2).

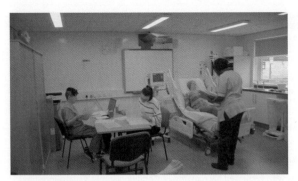

**Fig. 6.2** ■ An evening on call in progress.

# BRIEFING FOR AN INTERPROFESSIONAL LEARNING SIMULATION

Briefing for meaningful learning in IPL simulation should involve briefing both the faculty members and learners. Learners need to know the team they will be working alongside, and introductions should include establishing each other's professional background, level of skill, and previous experience of interprofessional simulation. As always, ground rules to promote safety of the learners should be agreed and adhered to. Section Briefing for Learners provides an overview of key points that should be addressed during the learners' briefing, contextualised to an IPL session.

## Briefing for Faculty

To promote consistency and parity in the learner experience, and for the purpose of quality assurance, a faculty meeting facilitates the opportunity to set the scene for the day. This should be a scheduled meeting which all faculty should be requested to attend, in advance of the session. This is an opportunity for team building and allows faculty to come together to discuss key concepts of the session. As cohesive facilitation and co-facilitation are aided by socialisation, we would encourage a 'coffee and conversation' approach to this. This approach will help faculty to feel at ease which will contribute to the development of partnership working and a shared mental model. It is important to include all faculty members (administration, technical, and debrief teams). As the coordinator of the session normally has responsibility for ensuring the smooth running of the simulation course overall, they should chair the faculty meeting at start of each session.

The following is an example of a faculty briefing checklist:

- Welcome and thank you for supporting the session.
- Provide an overview of the purpose of the session.
- Faculty introductions.
- Clarify different roles of the faculty.
- Explain programme for the day:
  - Walk through the programme timings.
  - Inform of refreshments and break times and areas.
- Ensure all faculty relevant paperwork is distributed to faculty.
- Inform faculty of communication system and strategy for the session.
- Access to patient systems and clinical guidelines.
- Session evaluation process for learners and faculty.
- Coordinator will be available for any questions.
- Allow questions from faculty.
- Final comments.

## Briefing for Learners

The facilitator should provide a brief overview of the format of the session, which aligns to the ILOs. In the case study example provided later, this included demonstration of clinical prioritisation and communication skills. There are two main components to the learners' briefing for an IPL simulation. Firstly, information relevant to the group as a whole should be provided. This should then be followed by information relevant to individual professions. We will draw on the example of our case study to illustrate this.

The following is an example of a learner briefing checklist:

- Welcome and housekeeping.
- Introductions & creating a safe psychological space.
- Brief overview of session.
- Focused ILOs for session.
- Explanation of how feedback will be given.

- Orientation to the learning environment and equipment.
- Introduction to technical support team.
- Signposting for pastoral support.
- Emphasise this is a learning opportunity and not a test.

Additional considerations for briefing in-situ simulation:

- Professional in charge of clinical area responsible for patient safety.
- The clinical space where simulation and debrief will occur.
- Fire exits and any expected drills.
- Location of toilets.
- Highlight where simulation signage is displayed (AV recording, etc).
- Simulated contact numbers to be used for clinical emergency call and paging displayed.
- The need to return the area ready for clinical use promptly.

## DELIVERING AN INTERPROFESSIONAL LEARNING SIMULATION

Precision is key and if the faculty are to gain, and maintain, a good reputation for their delivery of IPL, a key part of this is ensuring that the simulation runs to the planned schedule. Similarly, the strategy planned to terminate the simulation component should be made clear to the learner. This can take the form of a sound (e.g., a bell ringing) or the arrival of senior staff for the learner to handover to. In addition to reducing unnecessary stress for learners, this level of precision and organisation optimises the credibility of the faculty and/or simulation centre.

### Roles and Responsibility of Faculty

The faculty available to deliver an IPL simulation session can vary in terms of demographic and numbers, and it may be necessary for some of the team to adopt multiple roles. Table 6.7 provides a brief overview of

| TABLE 6.7 | |
|---|---|
| **Roles and Responsibilities of Faculty** | |
| **Faculty Member** | **Role During Delivery of Simulation** |
| Coordinator | ■ Responsible for ensuring the smooth running of the session. Including:<br>　■ Administration<br>　■ Timekeeping<br>　■ Leading the simulation faculty<br>　■ Explaining programme of events<br>　■ Managing flow of learners |
| Technicians | ■ Pre-programming scenario on manikin software<br>■ Audio-visual support<br>■ Troubleshooting technical problems<br>■ Ensuring adequate amount of equipment and consumables |
| Embedded professional | ■ Maintaining the immersion<br>■ Being familiar with the scenario to provide accurate information when this is requested<br>■ Assisting with patient assessments<br>■ Resetting the environment, ready for the next session or clinical use |
| Educator/Facilitator | ■ During simulation:<br>　■ Observing learners – does not intervene<br>　■ Marking feedback sheet, making written comments as observed<br>　■ Taking learner handover at the end of the simulation as next shift<br>■ Leading reflection, debrief, and learner's evaluation of the experience:<br>　■ Inviting learner's reflection on performance<br>　■ Using feedback form to provide constructive feedback<br>　■ Providing learner with copy of completed feedback form to facilitate personal reflection and future development<br>　■ Asking learners to complete post-session evaluation |

the roles and responsibilities of the team to help deliver a smooth-running IPL simulation and meaningful learning experience.

## Setting the Scene

The coordinator and facilitator work together in setting the scene, and immediately prior to beginning the immersive simulation, the facilitator should introduce the scenario by providing clear, succinct background information. Ideally, this should take the form of a verbal and printed handover, using a structured communication tool (e.g., SBAR). To confirm a shared mental model, the facilitator should confirm the learner's understanding of the scenario by inviting them to repeat it. This verifies that learners have heard the relevant details and, if required, provides the facilitator with an opportunity to rectify any misunderstandings. Learners should then be encouraged to ask any final questions.

Finally, in terms of a safe learning environment, it is worth reminding the learner that this is a simulation, which can be paused should they feel overwhelmed. When this happens, a facilitated learning conversation may be required where the learner should be encouraged to pause, breathe, think, and plan.

### The following is a pre-scenario checklist:

- Introduce the scenario.
- Ask learner to repeat.
- Allow for questions.
- Discuss time out strategy.

## Promoting Authenticity

Within the context of an interprofessional simulation, maintaining the immersion for all learners is key. With this in mind, it is important the simulation environment reflects the real health and care environment, which requires a degree of attention to detail. In addition to staff uniforms, documentation charts, sundries and consumables being authentic, an added dimension is to promote realistic timelines associated with any examinations and care delivered. This means when learners request investigations (e.g., blood samples) or interventions (e.g., insert PVC), a relevant period of time should lapse before disclosing results

(see Fidelity sections in Chapters 4 and 5). In addition to augmenting the authenticity of the simulation, this provides learners with the opportunity to process information and think before making their clinical decisions.

Another aspect to consider, relating to immersion and the authenticity of the simulation, is the clinical knowledge and skill level of the learner, who should not work above their level of clinical competence. This means they are required to escalate the care of the patient in the scenario, as the acuity changes. Having a communication system to contact senior colleagues available can minimise the risk of the learner feeling isolated or overwhelmed by their scenario. The senior colleague must be supportive and not obstructive.

## Maintaining the Flow and Integrity of the Simulation

Although our scenarios are written with set ILOs in mind, and we have strategies in place to guide the trajectory of the simulation, we cannot predict the learners' actions when they are immersed in the session. In situations where a scenario is going off track by a learner misdiagnosing or attempting treatment which, in reality, would be detrimental to the patient, the faculty must respond without compromising the flow and integrity of the simulation. Input from a well-briefed simulated patient or embedded professional (EP) can be invaluable in these circumstances. Any attempts at questionable interventions by the learner will form part of the profession specific debrief (see Learner Individual Debrief (Uniprofessional) section). It is worth trying to pre-empt some common requests the learners may make and draw up strategies as a team to address these during the faculty briefing session.

Similarly, the faculty debriefing session (see Faculty Debrief in Interprofessional Learning Simulation section) provides an ideal forum for faculty to reflect on the scenario(s), highlight issues where learners are going off track, and plan a way forward. It may be you need to follow the advice in Chapter 4 and consider adapting your scenario, but in situations where you are delivering a series of sessions to a large cohort of learners consecutively, there may not be the time for this. Some potential responses to help maintain the integrity of the simulation could be:

| Potential Learner Action | Response |
| --- | --- |
| Asks for blood results, ECGs, X-rays, that are not available | EP assumes these to be normal and informs the doctor. |
| Asks for additional investigations which are not relevant to the patient scenario | EP to state these will be organised, and you will inform them when this is done. |
| Wishes to initiate treatment or interventions which are potentially harmful to the patient | EP to advise that this would not be normal practice and they should seek advice from a senior medical colleague (offer the contact number). |
| Misdiagnoses acute coronary syndrome (ACS) for pericarditis | Simulated patient to state: 'this feels the same as when I had my heart attack.' |

## Terminating the Session

The coordinator should draw the simulation component to a clear conclusion, and the learner should be in no doubt that the immersion has ended. It is essential to allow all involved to decompress and proceed into the designated area for debriefing. It is useful for the facilitator responsible for delivering the feedback and debrief session to be in earshot of the learners as this is the time to capture the learner's immediate, true emotions after the event. These comments are like gold to the facilitator, as it is often an excellent opening gambit for the debrief.

## Additional Considerations for Delivering In-Situ Simulation

In the section on Planning an In-Situ Interprofessional Learning Simulation we advised conducting a robust risk assessment before the session. Although the risk assessment confirms the area is safe to deliver a teaching session, without compromising patient or staff

safety, it is worth noting this is only valid at the time the assessment was completed. The health and care environment is dynamic and patient acuity is prone to change; therefore, the coordinator should contact the area immediately before the planned session to confirm it is safe to start. The absolute priority will always be the safety of real patients.

Delivering in-situ simulation is stressful and intense for the clinical team and the simulation faculty. However, the benefits of these sessions in developing a cohesive team are invaluable to the delivery of safe and effective patient care. A balance is required between the opportunity to learn and clinical safety. This can be achieved through careful crafting of conceptual, physical, and psychological fidelity to enhance the capacity to learn (see Chapter 4) through immersion in an authentic environment, balanced with clinical risk, quality assurance, and clinical governance.

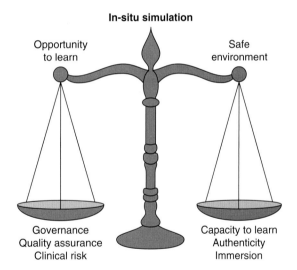

In-situ simulation

Opportunity to learn — Safe environment

Governance Quality assurance Clinical risk — Capacity to learn Authenticity Immersion

## Learner Well-Being

IPL simulation exercises can be an intense and stressful experience for learners, which has the potential to evoke emotions and generate questions relating to clinical care and the role of the team. Faculty should be sensitive to learners' non-verbal signs of stress and, if necessary, implement the strategy agreed earlier in the session, when setting the scene for the learners (see section on Setting the Scene). A key component to supporting learners is the presence of professional support from each discipline. In addition to offering pastoral support, this serves to enhance the credibility of the immersive simulation.

## DEBRIEFING AN INTERPROFESSIONAL LEARNING SIMULATION

Debriefing after the IPL simulation facilitates the deconstruction of the learning experience and supports the development of new knowledge for the learner. As with all debriefing in simulation, this involves a facilitative process whereby all learners are invited to contribute to the conversation about their experience. Key components include the ILOs, scenario objectives, and discussion points, ideally as identified by the learners. The facilitator guides the learning conversation using techniques for debriefing (see Chapters 3 and 5 for additional information on debriefing). However, as there is often lots of information to process when observing an IPL simulation, it may be useful to take notes during observation of the simulation, to inform the debrief discussion afterwards.

Depending upon the stage of the learners, the session aims, and the ILOs of the session, you may require a twofold approach to debriefing. This could take the form of an individual, uniprofessional approach initially, followed by an interprofessional debrief, where all professions involved in the exercise participate.

### Learner Individual Debrief (Uniprofessional)

A uniprofessional debrief should be facilitated by a simulation educator who is a subject matter expert in the same professional field as the learner. This allows learners to explore the application of their knowledge and understanding to the scenario(s) and provides an opportunity to address any questions which are at the forefront for students, and also to support in situations where crisis of confidence on the part of the learner may present, particularly in relation to their clinical ability. It also allows exploration and confirmation of the learner's underpinning knowledge and provides an opportunity for a concise, targeted teaching session to fill any knowledge gaps, if this is required (microteach). If gaps in knowledge are identified, the session should include a discussion focused on an action plan for learning.

A uniprofessional debrief can clear the learners mind, allowing them to fully engage in the interprofessional debrief without being preoccupied by questions they believe to be left unanswered from their own professional perspective. To standardise the information collected while observing the simulation, you may find it useful to develop a proforma to record notes. An example of one we have used can be found in Table 6.8.

### Time Out

Think about your planned IPL session and your ILOs and, with reference to these, draw up your own debriefing tool for your learners. Please note, it may be worth inviting each discipline to develop their own debriefing tool according to their individual ILOs.

### Learner Interprofessional Debrief

Facilitating the debriefing of an IPL simulation requires skill (ASPiH, 2017), and success relies on the ability of facilitators to interact and to direct learning for all professions involved (van Diggele et al., 2020). However, even the most experienced facilitators can find observing an IPL simulation challenging because of the amount of information which must be processed. Similar to the individual debrief, a strategy we have found useful in focusing the minds of the debriefing team, while observing the simulation, is to use an aide memoir. This helps generate a consistent approach and parity of learner experience. An example can be found in Table 6.9.

When the professions within the faculty mirror the professions of those learning, the credibility of the teaching team to deliver the session is enhanced, and learners can feel represented, meaning they are more likely to engage in the conversation. It is therefore essential to have an interprofessional debriefing team. From a faculty perspective, it would be challenging to completely appreciate the roles and expectations of other professions and, in this respect, the interprofessional approach to debriefing will serve

| TABLE 6.8 |
|---|
| **Evening on Call Individual Learner Debrief** |

Please circle the level attained by the learner using the scale below.

During the session, the learner:

1. Demonstrates ability to prioritise workload effectively, particularly in respect of emergency situations.

| Well below expectations for stage of learning | Below expectations for stage of learning | Meets expectations for stage of learning | Above expectations for stage of learning | Well above expectations for stage of learning |
|---|---|---|---|---|
| Comments | | | | |

2. Demonstrates the ability to communicate effectively with patients, colleagues, and other professionals.

| Well below expectations for stage of learning | Below expectations for stage of learning | Meets expectations for stage of learning | Above expectations for stage of learning | Well above expectations for stage of learning |
|---|---|---|---|---|
| Comments | | | | |

3. Carries out systematic ABCDE assessment of the sick patient.

| Well below expectations for stage of learning | Below expectations for stage of learning | Meets expectations for stage of learning | Above expectations for stage of learning | Well above expectations for stage of learning |
|---|---|---|---|---|
| Comments | | | | |

4. Recognises personal limitations, when appropriate communicates effectively with senior to ask advice re situation.

| Well below expectations for stage of learning | Below expectations for stage of learning | Meets expectations for stage of learning | Above expectations for stage of learning | Well above expectations for stage of learning |
|---|---|---|---|---|
| Comments | | | | |

5. Demonstrates ability to make effective clinical decisions.

| Well below expectations for stage of learning | Below expectations for stage of learning | Meets expectations for stage of learning | Above expectations for stage of learning | Well above expectations for stage of learning |
|---|---|---|---|---|
| Comments | | | | |

*Continued*

**TABLE 6.8 (Continued)**

**Evening on Call Individual Learner Debrief**

6. Demonstrates ability to document patient information.

| Well below expectations for stage of learning | Below expectations for stage of learning | Meets expectations for stage of learning | Above expectations for stage of learning | Well above expectations for stage of learning |
|---|---|---|---|---|
| Comments | | | | |

7. Can competently perform clinical skills as appropriate for level of learning.

| Well below expectations for stage of learning | Below expectations for stage of learning | Meets expectations for stage of learning | Above expectations for stage of learning | Well above expectations for stage of learning |
|---|---|---|---|---|
| Comments | | | | |

Personalised learner action plan (discuss with learner areas which require further support/review)

Learning Need:

| How will learning be achieved? (Please tick) | Online learning | Course attendance | Independent learning | Supervised clinical practice | Other (please specify) | How long will this take? |
|---|---|---|---|---|---|---|
| | | | | | | |

Reflection on learning

**What was the session? (What?)**

**What did you understand from the learning? (So what?)**

**How will you apply this learning to your practice? (Now what?)**

Adapted from Rolfe, G., Freshwater, D., Jasper, M., 2001. *Critical reflection in nursing and the helping professions: A user's guide.* Basingstoke: Palgrave Macmillan.

## TABLE 6.9
### Interprofessional Debrief Tool

While technical skills for practice are easily taught, the intricacies of non-technical skills (NTS) are more difficult to acquire. As the most common cause of adverse events in practice is a consequence of deficiencies in NTS, these are vital in the promotion of patient safety.

This IPL session is designed to afford learners the opportunity to work as part of a team and experience first-hand the role NTS play in the coordinated, safe, effective management of a patient.

Please circle the level attained by the learner using the scale below.

1. **Task management:** planning & preparing, prioritising, providing & maintaining standards, identifying & utilising resources.

| Well below expectations for stage of learning | Below expectations for stage of learning | Meets expectations for stage of learning | Above expectations for stage of learning | Well above expectations for stage of learning |
|---|---|---|---|---|
| Comments | | | | |

2. **Situation awareness:** gathering information, recognising and understanding, anticipating standards, identifying & utilising resources.

| Well below expectations for stage of learning | Below expectations for stage of learning | Meets expectations for stage of learning | Above expectations for stage of learning | Well above expectations for stage of learning |
|---|---|---|---|---|
| Comments | | | | |

3. **Communication:** strategies used, effectiveness of these.

| Well below expectations for stage of learning | Below expectations for stage of learning | Meets expectations for stage of learning | Above expectations for stage of learning | Well above expectations for stage of learning |
|---|---|---|---|---|
| Comments | | | | |

4. **Decision making:** identifying options, balancing risks and selecting options, re-evaluating.

| Well below expectations for stage of learning | Below expectations for stage of learning | Meets expectations for stage of learning | Above expectations for stage of learning | Well above expectations for stage of learning |
|---|---|---|---|---|
| Comments | | | | |

5. **Team working:** coordinating activities with team, exchanging information, using authority and assertiveness, assessing capabilities, supporting others.

| Well below expectations for stage of learning | Below expectations for stage of learning | Meets expectations for stage of learning | Above expectations for stage of learning | Well above expectations for stage of learning |
|---|---|---|---|---|
| Comments | | | | |

to enrich the learning environment. As facilitators of learning, all disciplines have valuable contributions to make to the learning experience in the form of subject-specific knowledge, which will be beneficial to both learners and faculty members from across disciplines.

The aims of IPL are to provide an opportunity for learners to develop insight across a range of professional roles, and also to gain valuable experience working as part of a team. The debrief enables learners to reflect on what the other professions bring to the team, and how they all work together. Learners can develop an understanding of what constitutes an effective team, as well as their individual contribution within the team, to enhance the delivery of safe, effective, person-centred care. Collaboration within the team will improve with increased knowledge of colleague's roles, generating a culture of respect which can transfer to practice. Indeed, IPL simulation has been identified as a strategy to build positive attitudes on learning together and professional identity (Burford et al., 2020). With this in mind, we would always encourage debrief facilitators to end the session by asking learners to share their 'Take Home Message', outlining what will they take into their own practice as a result of this IPL simulation experience.

Chapter 3 presents a more detailed account of debriefing strategies. Taking into consideration the evidence-based tips for debriefing (Ross, 2021), these have been applied to IPL in Box 6.1.

## Faculty Debrief in Interprofessional Learning Simulation

It is good practice to conduct a post-session debrief for faculty, where open and transparent discussion can take place. In addition to providing a forum for faculty to decompress, opinions and ideas to augment the learner and faculty experience can be shared, and scenarios can be fine-tuned. From a personal development perspective, one-to-one faculty debrief sessions can facilitate the opportunity for feedback, allowing faculty to reflect on their own experience and performance. Thereafter, areas requiring support for further development can be identified and action plans created. This is referred to as the meta-debrief (see Chapter 3). Both the group and individual approaches to

faculty debrief will serve as strategies to promote quality assurance.

## EVALUATION

Evaluation of sessions adds to information gathered as part of the learner and faculty debrief, which contributes further to the quality assurance process. There are a number of ways to gather information relating to the learner and faculty experience to inform future practice sessions, and this will be discussed in greater depth as part of Chapter 9. Anonymity is, however, key to promoting engagement and honesty in the evaluation process and can be achieved via either online or paper evaluations. Examples of learner and faculty evaluations can be found in Tables 6.10 and 6.11.

### Time Out

Using the template as a guide, now consider the questions you would ask to evaluate your sessions.

## CASE STUDY: AN EVENING ON CALL SIMULATION

Earlier in the chapter we provided a synopsis of our IPL simulation 'An Evening on Call' (see Planning an In-Situ Interprofessional Learning Simulation). The simulation was designed to provide undergraduate students with the opportunity to experience working as part of an interprofessional team to emulate their roles within a medical unit and prepare them for their pending posts in healthcare. The ILOs met the needs of all professions involved in the simulation. The role of medical and nursing students was to assess patients in a dynamic clinical environment. Using an ABCDE approach to assessment, they then prioritised patient care according to acuity. Then, recognising their own clinical limitations, learners escalated care, when appropriate, to senior colleagues. The role of the pharmacy students was to support and offer advice to medical and nursing staff with clinical decisions, and treatment relating to medicine management, prescribing, and administration.

## BOX 6.1

## APPLICATION OF ROSS (2021) TWELVE TIPS TO INTERPROFESSIONAL LEARNING DEBRIEF

| Tip | Applied to Interprofessional Learning Debriefing |
| --- | --- |
| 1. Train the facilitators | Ensure the facilitators delivering the interprofessional learning (IPL) debriefing sessions have participated in an IPL workshop for this, and novice debriefers are supported. |
| 2. Ensure that facilitators observe the simulation | Ensure the role of the debriefer is protected, and their sole purpose is to observe the simulation to effectively facilitate the debrief. This requires a team approach with team members allocated to their specific roles. To help the debriefer remain focused throughout their observation of the simulation, templates may be useful for taking notes. |
| 3. Select the most appropriate timing for the debriefing | Within the context of IPL simulation, there may be the need for a twofold approach to debriefing: uniprofessional alongside the more collaborative approach of an interprofessional debrief. |
| 4. Conduct the debriefing in a safe environment | Peppering debriefing facilitators among the learners is key to preventing a 'teacher–learner' approach and will aid free flow of discussion. It is a good idea to ensure facilitators are in clear line of site of each other to aid co-facilitation. |
| 5. Tie the debriefing to the learning objectives | Refer back to the simulation and learner's agreed ILOs during the debrief. The facilitators may use these to generate discussion. By including the learner's ILOs for the session, learners have a degree of ownership, and their contribution is valued. |
| 6. Set the stage for the learners at the start of the debriefing | Promote a culture of safety and remind learners this is a safe space to practice in a mistake-forgiving environment and we will all learn from each other. |
| 7. Ensure there is a shared understanding of events | A recap of events can help to promote a shared mental model. You can invite any learner to volunteer their perception of the simulation event. |
| 8. Structure the debriefing using a framework or model | The debriefing tool to be used should be presented and agreed as part of the faculty briefing. |
| 9. Ask open-ended questions | While open-ended questions facilitate discussion, a word of caution in an IPL simulation. By nature, IPL simulations can evoke feelings of vulnerability among learners and asking 'Why?' can be perceived as confrontational. Choose your language wisely to promote a non-judgmental approach. |
| 10. Allow the learners to drive the discussion | The microteach is a useful tool to enable facilitators and learners to remain focused on the key points of the debrief. Avoid too much anecdotal, non-contextualised discussion. Remember the learners' voices should be dominant in the debrief. |
| 11. Recognize the importance of non-verbal communication | Useful for facilitating the debrief as a co-debriefer. When there is more than one facilitator, strategic positioning in the debrief environment means all facilitators should be in eyeline of each other and still be able to view all learners. |
| 12. Use the silence | Use silence with purpose. It will not last long following an IPL simulation. |

Ross, S., 2021. Twelve tips for effective simulation debriefing: A research-based approach. Medical Teacher, 43(6), pp.642-645.

| TABLE 6.10 | | | | | |
|---|---|---|---|---|---|
| **Learner Evaluation Form** | | | | | |

Please circle the relevant number and PRINT comments

| | *Strongly Agree* | | | | *Strongly Disagree* |
|---|---|---|---|---|---|
| I found the session enjoyable. | 1 | 2 | 3 | 4 | 5 |
| I learned new skills regarding prioritisation of duties. | 1 | 2 | 3 | 4 | 5 |
| I learned new skills regarding communication with various members of a clinical team. | 1 | 2 | 3 | 4 | 5 |
| The session was well organised. | 1 | 2 | 3 | 4 | 5 |
| The faculty was well-informed and enthusiastic about the session. | 1 | 2 | 3 | 4 | 5 |
| The venue of the session was fit for purpose. | 1 | 2 | 3 | 4 | 5 |
| The session will be beneficial in my junior post qualification year and beyond. | 1 | 2 | 3 | 4 | 5 |
| I would recommend this session be part of all students Preparation for Practice blocks. | 1 | 2 | 3 | 4 | 5 |

| Comments: |
|---|
| Please indicate any areas you particularly enjoyed/found valuable in the session |
| Please indicate any areas you didn't enjoy/didn't find as beneficial |

| TABLE 6.11 | | |
|---|---|---|
| **Faculty Evaluation Form** | | |

| Name: | Date: | Venue: |
|---|---|---|
| | | |

To improve the programme, we would be grateful for your opinions and suggestions. Where appropriate, please circle Yes or No and provide comments.

| 1. Was the quantity and quality of the information you received adequate? | Yes | No |
|---|---|---|
| **Comments** | | |

| 2. Did any issues arise that we could have been better prepared for? | Yes | No |
|---|---|---|
| **Comments** | | |

| TABLE 6.11 (Continued) | | |
|---|---|---|
| **Faculty Evaluation Form** | | |
| 3. In your opinion, was the session beneficial to the candidate? | Yes | No |
| **Comments** | | |
| 4. Do you have any comments regarding the structure and timings of the session? | Yes | No |
| **Comments** | | |
| 5. In your opinion, what was the least important/ beneficial aspect of the session? | | |
| **Comments** | | |
| 6. Do you feel the students were appropriately challenged? | Yes | No |
| **Comments** | | |
| 7. Was it a realistic representation of clinical experience? | Yes | No |
| **Comments** | | |
| 8. Was there a sufficient spread of pathophysiologies for a 1-hour session? | | |
| **Comments** | | |
| 9. Do you feel documentation was covered sufficiently? | Yes | No |
| **Comments** | | |
| **Any Other Comments** | | |

## CASE STUDY

### An Evening on Call Simulation

*SESSION AIM*

To provide learners with the opportunity, through an immersive simulation experience, to understand their critical role within an interprofessional team and to safely prioritise care for a group of patients.

*INTENDED LEARNING OBJECTIVES*

*By the end of the session students will be able to*:

- Use a systematic ABCDE (Airway, Breathing, Circulation, Disability, Exposure) assessment when examining a patient **(apply)**
- Demonstrate the use of clinical decision-making skills to prioritise workload **(apply)**
- Recognise indications for escalation of patient's care to relevant colleagues **(knowledge)**
- Demonstrate effective communication skills within an interprofessional team **(apply)**
- Apply the SBAR (Situation, Background, Assessment, Recommendation) tool as a communication strategy **(apply)**
- Demonstrate safe, accurate, appropriate medication prescribing and administration **(knowledge)**
- Demonstrate safe, accurate documentation skills **(knowledge)**
- Interpret, analyse, and appropriately respond to results of investigations **(analyse)**

- Demonstrate effective time management skills **(apply)**
- Demonstrate leadership skills through the safe and appropriate delegation of tasks **(apply)**
- Demonstrate personal situational awareness and recognise own limitations **(self-awareness knowledge)**

*TIMETABLE*

The timetable shown in Table 6.12 reflects one student's experience of the evening on call simulation from briefing through to debriefing. However, as the session ran concurrently, when one group reached the halfway point of the immersion, a second group would arrive for briefing (Table 6.13).

*ROLES AND RESPONSIBILITIES OF FACULTY*

As with all IPL simulation, it was essential to clearly define the roles and responsibilities of all faculty members to ensure an authentic experience for the learners. Inspired by the previous work of Swann et al. (2008), McGlynn et al. (2012) adapted and developed an IPL experience in a health board in Central Scotland for an interprofessional group of undergraduate healthcare students. This required an interprofessional faculty and the roles and responsibilities outlined in Table 6.14 are reflective of the faculty involved in the delivery of the NHSL *evening on call* programme.

| TABLE 6.12 | | |
|---|---|---|
| **Overview of Student Session Plan** | | |
| Session | Time | Activity |
| 1 | 15 mins | Introductions, aim & learning outcomes, and format of the session |
| 2 | 15 mins | Orientation to geographical layout of clinical area and contact numbers of colleagues (telephones and pagers)<br>SBAR handover from previous shift |
| 3 | 60 mins | Immersive simulation |
| 4 | 30 mins | Hot debrief (uniprofessional) |
| | 30 mins | Interprofessional debrief |

| TABLE 6.13 | | | | | | | | | |
|---|---|---|---|---|---|---|---|---|---|
| **Student Flow** | | | | | | | | | |
| 0900 | 0930 | 1000 | 1030 | 1100 | 1130 | 1200 | 1230 | 1300 | |
| Group 1 Briefing | Group 1 Immersion | | Group 1 Hot Debrief | Group 1 IP Debrief | | | | | |
| | | Group 2 Briefing | Group 2 Immersion | | Group 2 Hot Debrief | Group 2 IP Debrief | | | |
| | | | | Group 3 Briefing | Group 3 Immersion | | Group 3 Hot Debrief | Group 3 IP Debrief | |

| TABLE 6.14 | | | |
|---|---|---|---|
| **Evening on Call Faculty Roles and Responsibilities** | | | |
| Faculty | Pre-simulation | During Simulation | Post-simulation |
| **Coordinator** | Ensures the smooth running of the session.<br>**Faculty:**<br>■ Chair Faculty Meeting:<br>■ Distribution of paperwork to faculty.<br>■ Explain programme for the day.<br>■ Clarify different roles of the faculty.<br>**Learners:**<br>■ Meet learners.<br>■ Orientate learners to simulation area.<br>■ Explain paging system.<br>■ Explain format of the simulation.<br>■ Introduce to facilitators. | ■ Timekeeping<br>■ Inform learners and facilitators when the immersion component is complete. | ■ Direct learners and facilitators to debrief area.<br>■ Hold stock of paperwork and props for replenishing purposes.<br>■ Ensure session documentation is completed and filed appropriately.<br>■ Remind learners and faculty to complete simulation experience evaluation. |
| **Role of the Educator/ Facilitator** | ■ Provide printed and verbal handover (SBAR).<br>■ Allow for questions. | ■ Fully immersed in the simulation.<br>■ Observe learners and do not intervene.<br>■ Take handover from learner at the end of the immersion. | ■ Facilitate reflection and a structured debrief.<br>■ Provide learners with written feedback on their performance.<br>■ Ask learner to complete programme evaluation. |
| **Embedded professional** | ■ Be cognisant of the patients in their ward. | ■ Know which patients have been handed over to the on-call doctor.<br>■ Know the script to maintain the immersion of the simulation.<br>■ Assist Dr to perform patient assessments and provide accurate information. | ■ Reset the simulation environment. |
| **Role of the on-call Senior Colleague** | ■ Fully understand the scenarios.<br>■ Be prepared to give advice and answer questions.<br>■ Carry phone or page. | ■ Be present within the environment.<br>■ Be supportive of junior colleagues.<br>■ Be prepared to participate if learner's psychological safety appears compromised. | ■ Facilitate one-to-one feedback.<br>■ Address gaps in learner's knowledge.<br>■ Deliver microteach as appropriate. |

# TOP TIPS FOR INTERPROFESSIONAL LEARNING SIMULATION-BASED EDUCATION

| Top Tip | Guidance |
|---|---|
| ■ **Begin planning early** | Scope out the breadth of professions required and their availability to participate. |
| | Organise a planning meeting at least 6 months in advance to agree and set intended learning objectives (ILOs). |
| | Agree tasks, allocate responsibility and set timelines. |
| ■ **Book and confirm the venue** | This can be one of the more challenging aspects and requires forethought. Considerations need to be given to the space available, timing of session, equipment required, and faculty. |
| ■ **A collaborative faculty approach is key** | This ensures representation of all professional groups within the simulation faculty and role-models the interprofessional working we are trying to emulate. This facilitates a collaborative approach to the planning, delivery, and evaluation of any interprofessional learning (IPL) simulation. |
| | ILOs should be relevant to all learners and involve key representatives from each profession. Consideration should be given to the contribution of each professional group in terms of uniprofessional knowledge and skills, and the cross professional learning which is likely to occur. |

| Top Tip | Guidance |
|---|---|
| ■ **Engage with learners in advance of the simulation activity** | Provide learners with access to the ILOs, and any preparatory material in advance of the session. |
| ■ **Prepare the learners well** | It is important to recognise the importance of the briefing session which is essential to adequately prepare learners. This provides an opportunity to answer any questions and promote a psychologically safe environment. |
| ■ **Promote authenticity: Balance learner numbers to reflect clinical practice** | The IPL simulation is augmented when staff ratios broadly match the clinical team composition and promotes authentic teamwork within the simulation session. By preventing an imbalance in professional representation, the risk of learners feeling isolated is minimised. |
| ■ **Do not allow learners to become distracted at the end of the simulation** | Learners often try to tidy away equipment immediately after the simulation, but it is advisable to discourage this as it acts as a diversion and can deflect from the immediate decompression from the experience. Have faculty on standby to reset and direct the learners to the debriefing area. |
| ■ **Ensure time for post-course debrief** | This is good practice to ensure the session meets the needs of all professions equally and allows further faculty development needs to be identified. |
| **Allocate time for evaluation** | Plan in advance the evaluation strategy from both the learners' and facilitators' perspective. |

| Top Tip | Guidance |
|---|---|
| *Additional Considerations for In-Situ Interprofessional Learning Simulation* | |
| ▪ **Plan and prepare** | Meet with the lead/link person from the department to discuss and agree a suitable plan. |
| ▪ **Scope the clinical area** | This is crucial. You may find simulation equipment requires to be tested in the clinical area to ensure functionality. |
| ▪ **Choose an optimum time** | Identify a time when the clinical area is least likely to be under high clinical pressures. |
| ▪ **Ensure a risk assessment is in place** | This allows a clear process to ensure the clinical area is not compromised and establish clear plans to stop the simulation if the safety of real patients could become compromised. |
| ▪ **Share that IPL simulation is happening with others** | This might be via local daily email briefs, or displaying signage within the clinical area so other staff, patients, and relatives can see that an IPL simulation is taking place. |
| ▪ **Evaluate and share any learning** | Share the learning from the session by providing a written commentary to the department and relevant senior management teams. This is particularly useful if the simulation has highlighted latent threats to patient safety. |
| ▪ **Plan for the future** | Highlight staff from the area who have the potential to develop as simulation educators. This will facilitate future in-situ IPL sessions whenever opportunities arise. |

## SUMMARY

SBE is a powerful way to facilitate IPL. With the increasing recognition that this is a vital part of training, more thought has to be given in relation to how we can make this more normal and more efficacious to deliver. Widespread recognition that IPL is important is in itself a step forward. Educators must therefore build on relationships locally between teams from various health and care professions to decide what works for them in each context. There has to be engagement from across all levels of learner to foster an environment that will allow teams to test their ideas. It is vital that all learning is shared to help the wider simulation community progress and influence those at organisational and national levels. This will support development and implementation of authentic SBE.

## REFERENCES

Association for Simulation Practice in Healthcare (ASPiH), 2017. Simulation Based Education in Healthcare: Standards Framework and Guidance. Available at: https://aspih.org.uk/wp-content/uploads/2017/07/standards-framework.pdf.

Attoe, C., Lavelle, M., Sherwali, S., Rimes, K., Jabur, Z., 2018. Student interprofessional mental health simulation (SIMHS): evaluating the impact on medical and nursing students, and clinical psychology trainees. The Journal of Mental Health Training, Education and Practice 14 (1), 46–58.

Burford, B., Greig, P., Kelleher, M., Merriman, C., Platt, A., Richards, E., et al., 2020. Effects of a single interprofessional simulation session on medical and nursing students' attitudes toward interprofessional learning and professional identity: a questionnaire study. BMC Medical Education 20 (1), 1–11.

Carmela, R., Erica, B., Chiara, A., Silvia, C., Eleonora, G., Barisone, M., et al., 2022. The impact of an interprofessional simulation-based education intervention in healthy ageing: a quasi-experimental study. Clinical Simulation in Nursing 64, 1–9.

Centre for the Advancement of Interprofessional Education (CAIPE), 2021. Interprofessional Education Handbook: For Educators and Practitioners Incorporating Integrated Care and Values-Based Practice, (Ford, J., Gray, R.) [Online]. Accessed 10th Oct 2022. Available from: https://www.caipe.org/resources/publications/caipe-publications/caipe-2021-a-new-caipe-interprofessional-education-handbook-2021-ipe-incorporating-values-based-practice-ford-j-gray-r.

Charles, S., Koehn, M.L., 2020. Logistics in simulation-based interprofessional education. In: Comprehensive Healthcare Simulation: InterProfessional Team Training and Simulation. Springer, New York, NY, pp. 135–155.

Collins, K., Layne, K.C., Andrea, C., Perry, L.A., 2021. The impact of interprofessional simulation experiences in occupational and physical therapy education: a qualitative study. Cadernos Brasileiros de Terapia Ocupacional 29.

Dharamsi, A., Hayman, K., Yi, S., Chow, R., Yee, C., Gaylord, E., et al., 2020. Enhancing departmental preparedness for COVID-19 using rapid-cycle in-situ simulation. Journal of Hospital Infection 105 (4), 604–607.

Goolsarran, N., Hamo, C.E., Lane, S., Frawley, S., Lu, W.H., 2018. Effectiveness of an interprofessional patient safety team-based learning simulation experience on healthcare professional trainees. BMC Medical Education 18 (1), 1–8.

Goulding, M.H., Graham, L., Chorney, D., Rajendram, R., 2020. The use of interprofessional simulation to improve collaboration and problem solving among undergraduate BHSc medical laboratory science and BScN nursing students. Canadian Journal of Medical Laboratory Science 82 (2), 25–33.

Gros, E., Shi, R., Hasty, B., Anderson, T., Schmiederer, I., Roman-Micek, T., et al., 2021. In situ interprofessional operating room simulations: Empowering learners in crisis resource management principles. Surgery 170 (2), 432–439.

Holmes, C., Mellanby, E., 2022. Debriefing strategies for interprofessional simulation—a qualitative study. Advances in Simulation 7 (1), 1–19.

INACSL Standards Committee, 2016. Standards of best practice: simulation standard VIII: simulation-enhanced interprofessional education (Sim-IPE). Clinical Simulation in Nursing 12 (S), S34–S38.

Kleib, M., Jackman, D., Duarte-Wisnesky, U., 2021. Interprofessional simulation to promote teamwork and communication between nursing and respiratory therapy students: a mixed-method research study. Nurse Education Today 99,104816.

Lee, W., Kim, M., Kang, Y., Lee, Y.J., Kim, S.M., Lee, J., et al., 2020. Nursing and medical students' perceptions of an interprofessional simulation-based education: a qualitative descriptive study. Korean Journal of Medical Education 32 (4), 317.

McGlynn, M.C., Scott, H.R., Thomson, C., Peacock, S., Paton, C., 2012. How we equip undergraduates with prioritisation skills using simulated teaching scenarios. Medical Teacher 34 (7), 526–529.

McGregor, C.A., Paton, C., Thomson, C., Chandratilake, M., Scott, H., 2012. Preparing medical students for clinical decision making: a pilot study exploring how students make decisions and the perceived impact of a clinical decision making teaching intervention. Medical Teacher 34 (7), e508–e517.

Murray, M., 2021. The impact of interprofessional simulation on readiness for interprofessional learning in health professions students. Teaching and Learning in Nursing 16 (3), 199–204.

Rolfe, G., Freshwater, D., Jasper, M., 2001. Critical Reflection in Nursing and the Helping Professions: A User's Guide. Palgrave Macmillan, Basingstoke.

Ross, S., 2021. Twelve tips for effective simulation debriefing: A research-based approach. Medical Teacher, 43(6), pp.642–645.

Shi, R., Marin-Nevarez, P., Hasty, B., Roman-Micek, T., Hirx, S., Anderson, T., et al., 2021. Operating room in situ interprofessional simulation for improving communication and teamwork. Journal of Surgical Research 260, 237–244.

SSH and NLN, 2013. International education and healthcare simulation symposium. Available at: https://www.nln.org/docs/default-source/uploadedfiles/professional-development-programs/white-paper-symposium-ipe-in-healthcare-simulation-2013-pdf.pdf?sfvrsn=d608da0d_0.

Swann, R., Richardson, D., Wardle, J., Metcalf, J., 2008. 'Hard day's night'–an undergraduate interprofessional key skills training session. The Clinical Teacher 5 (2), 113–118.

Tallentire, V.R., Kerins, J., McColgan-Smith, S., Power, A., Stewart, F., Mardon, J., 2022. Exploring the impact of interprofessional simulation on the professional relationships of trainee pharmacists and medical students: a constructivist interview study. International Journal of Healthcare Simulation 2 (1), 1–11.

Tilley, C.P., Roitman, J., Zafra, K.P., Brennan, M., 2021. Real-time, simulation-enhanced interprofessional education in the care of older adults with multiple chronic comorbidities: a utilization-focused evaluation. Mhealth 7.

van Diggele, C., Roberts, C., Burgess, A., Mellis, C., 2020. Interprofessional education: tips for design and implementation. BMC Medical Education 20 (2), 1–6.

WHO, 2010. Framework for Action on Interprofessional Education and Collaborative Practice. http://aspih.org.uk/wp-content/uploads/2017/07/standards-framework.pdf. (Accessed 2022).

# 7

# LARGE GROUP SIMULATION

ELIZABETH SIMPSON ■ GAYLE ANN MACKIE

*Simulation for the masses, not masses of simulation.*
*Brown, Morse and Morrison, 2016*

## CHAPTER OUTLINE

INTRODUCTION

BACKGROUND

CONTEXT

PLANNING

BRIEFING

DELIVERY

CASE STUDY: LARGE GROUP SIMULATION

LARGE GROUP SIMULATION ON A BUDGET

TOP TIPS FOR LARGE GROUP SIMULATION

SUMMARY

## OBJECTIVES

*This chapter should support the reader to develop an understanding of the:*

- Challenges and benefits to large group simulation.
- Processes involved in planning, delivering, and evaluating large group simulation.
- Practicalities involved in large group simulation, through a case study.
- Use of participant response systems to promote learner engagement.

## KEY TERMS

Large scale simulation

Large audience simulation

Large group simulation

Mass simulation

Participant Response Systems (PRS)

Audience Response Systems (ARS)

Student Response Systems (SRS) Background

## INTRODUCTION

This chapter will consider an overview of the current challenges faced as part of contemporary healthcare delivery. There will be consideration of the role of large group simulation in developing the skills and behaviours required by health and care professionals. A definition of large group simulation will be provided, alongside the theory of learner engagement in the large group environment, exploring the role of response systems to promote this. Drawing on our experiences of planning, delivering, and evaluating a large group simulation exercise, practical advice will be presented, including the roles and responsibilities of the various faculty members. Finally, the chapter will present strategies to deliver large group simulation, particularly when faced with constraint on budget.

## BACKGROUND

While it is accepted across health and care disciplines that the development of non-technical skills and an awareness of human factors are essential aspects of patient safety, the logistics of teaching can be challenging. Professional regulation of health and care undergraduate courses means that newly registered practitioners qualify with a relatively broad range of practical skills, and often with sound theoretical knowledge of medical conditions. However, opportunities to apply critical thinking to practice can sometimes be limited (Harper et al., 2021). Within the United Kingdom, and in the undergraduate context, this could perhaps be attributed to increasing student populations and the associated increasing placement capacity demands which stem from this, effectively reducing opportunities to develop the necessary clinical decision-making skills. The fear and anxiety which can stem from the lack of opportunity to develop these clinical decision-making skills has been previously discussed by Rhodes and Curran (2005). At that time, they related this fear and anxiety to the undergraduates' lack of experience and preparedness for the clinical environment.

Within the post-registration context, the development of these skills is dependent on exposure to clinical and/or caring situations, sound educational support in practice as these situations occur, and opportunities for continuing professional development (CPD). As part of this, there has been an increasing recognition that an essential characteristic of the contemporary health and care professional is their capacity to make sound clinical judgements. And in fact, Benner (1982) presented the theory of novice to expert, acknowledging the significance of skill acquisition in developing these clinical judgement skills. Despite this, it is important to recognise that skill acquisition is a continuous process (Rhodes and Curran, 2005). Therefore, the development and implementation of simulations which include both technical and non-technical skills may be a partial solution, mainly as these will offer opportunities for critical thinking in a safe, practically focused situation, increasing knowledge and clinical judgement skills as part of this (Hope, Garside and Prescott, 2011).

We know that learners welcome active learning which is engaging. When they are involved, their learning experience is improved, the application of theory to practice is addressed, and information is retained (Moyer, 2016). Simulation-based education (SBE) is the ideal vehicle for active learning and, in addition to learning skills and procedures, it enables the development of problem-solving, critical thinking, clinical judgement, and clinical decision-making skills. When facilitated by a subject matter expert and role model, SBE can also improve confidence and competence. However, despite these well-recorded benefits of SBE, it also has a reputation for being labour and resource intensive (Dufrene and Young, 2014). When added to an already intensive curricula, which is pressurised as a consequence of time constraints, this presents a considerable challenge to the simulation educator. There is therefore an argument that the answer could be large group simulation. This argument is based on the premise that large group simulation can optimise time resources in high content load curricula (Moyer, 2016) and it is an effective alternative to the more didactic approach of lectures (Rode, Callihan and Barnes, 2016).

Our challenge is therefore to be creative and transform the normally passive learning atmosphere of the traditional lecture theatre or classroom environment into an engaging arena of participation and active learning. By so doing, we can address the issue of parity in the learning experience, which is often a source of learner dissatisfaction, particularly with large cohorts of learners being taught by a team of educators. Learners welcome methods that promote standardisation of the learning experience (Alhoqail and Badr, 2010), which can be achieved when presenting the simulation to the large group, simultaneously. We are in the midst of change within SBE as the latest advancement in simulation technology and the introduction of wireless systems allows more freedom of movement of manikins, equipment, and audio-visual (AV) systems. Therefore, as simulation educators, we are only restricted by our imagination and creativity. For those reading this chapter and thinking large group simulation is only possible with high-fidelity, top of the range equipment, be assured that this is not the case. This chapter will also present ways to achieve large group simulation with smaller budgets.

## CONTEXT

You may question why we would even consider delivering simulation to a large group when it appears to contradict the underpinning concept of SBE, which is normally delivered to small groups in a space where learners can feel safe in a cocoon of support. However, when faced with large cohorts of students, ensuring parity in the learner experience is a challenge, and large group simulation offers a potential solution. Furthermore, as the global pandemic introduced the need for more creativity, large group simulation is easily adaptable to remote learning.

Moving forward in this chapter, large group simulation will be interpreted and explored in the context of SBE with a large audience. For example, it could be within the lecture theatre environment where a simulated case study can unfold before a participating audience. This specific context, combined with the use of strategies to engage learners such as individual voting systems (response systems) (Brown, Morse and Morrison, 2016) or TAG team simulation (Fig. 7.1), where the audience provide constructive feedback on a specific component of the simulation (Levett-Jones et al., 2015; Levett-Jones et al., 2017), will form the basis for learning. As the delivery of large group simulation also requires an understanding of the practicalities of organising these events, strategies for success will be outlined, and the roles of the simulation faculty will also be considered.

### Theory of Educational Engagement and Interaction

*I hear, I know. I see, I remember. I do, I understand.*
*Confucius*

Effective learning will occur when learners are actively involved in an environment which promotes and values interactions between learners and educators (Durning and Artino, 2011). It could be argued this is easier to achieve within small group simulations. In these situations, the educator can gauge students' understanding; this is important as achieving meaningful interactions between students and educators within the large group setting can be challenging (Jain and Farley, 2012; Fry, Ketteridge, and Marshall, 2015). For large groups of learners, it

T = Theatrical, embracing the dramatic contribution of acting to education
A = Applied and directly relevant to clinical practice
G = Guided by a 'director' and 'narrator' who facilitate the learning experience
T = Tactical and strategically designed to achieve pre-defined learning outcomes
E = Engaging through immersion of participants and observers in authentic learning experiences
A = Active involvement in dynamic and unfolding simulation experiences
M = Meaningful, memorable, and designed to empower learners to become agents of change

Fig. 7.1 ■ Tag team. (From Levett-Jones T, Dwyer T, Reid-Searl K., Heaton L, Flenady T, Applegarth J, Guinea S, Andersen P. 2017. Preparing undergraduate students for the workforce in the context of patient safety through innovative simulation – Facilitator Guide Rockhampton: Central Queensland University.)

can be challenging to interpret whether or not each individual is achieving the required learning. There is therefore a risk of leaving weaker students behind if learning is just assumed to have taken place prior to moving on to more complex concepts (Connor, 2009). In recognising this potential pitfall, Connor (2009) was instrumental in the introduction of response systems to the lecture theatre environment to allow for real-time feedback. To put this into context, think about how often you have asked a question in a session with multiple learners, received an answer from one or two, and then moved on. In this situation there is little or no evidence that all learners have grasped what is being taught, or that all learners have reached the same conclusion when asked the question.

The term *student engagement* is used often in the literature, but it seems this sometimes relates to whether the learner is paying attention (Biggs and Tang, 2007). Student engagement was described by Barkley (2010) as the *intersection* between motivation and active learning (Fig. 7.2). Active learning will be discussed in more detail in the following sections, but firstly we must consider our learners' 'motivation' to learn if the desired outcome is effective engagement. Biggs and Tang (2007) suggest that the role of facilitators of learning is to adopt a teaching approach which is designed to motivate learners. Within the context of health and care disciplines, motivation to learn could be rooted in the duty bound, ethical obligation to *do no harm* associated with the Hippocratic Oath. Therefore, it is

feasible to suggest that health and care professionals inherently want to do the best for those in their care, and for some this may be motivation enough to learn. However, it is also important to recognise that career progression normally aligns with the gradual growth and development of clinical judgment skills. We also need to consider how if we 'don't know what we don't know', we will then reach the realisation that there is learning which we must achieve. In this situation, it may be that a combination of working alongside role models in practice and fear of potentially doing harm to those in our care may be motivating factors. Either way, realisation that learning is required, and thereafter motivation to learn, particularly when this will improve clinical skills and the ability to deliver safe, effective, person-centred care, tends to present in learners within the health and care profession.

Having established that both a realisation that learning is required and the motivation to learn must first exist, the next stage is to consider strategies to promote active learning to truly engage learners. In our large group simulation, active learning was clearly being undertaken by the small team of students delivering care to the patient as part of the immersive simulation, but our challenge was to encourage active participation by the audience. The audience were actively involved by the use of TurningPoint Polling, a form of response system which displays multiple choice questions for the audience to answer in real time. Responses were recorded, immediately analysed, the correct answer was given, and an explanation of this was provided. Response systems are not a new concept with Kay and LeSage (2009) reporting that they have been in use since early 1966. For the purpose of this chapter, we will refer to them as response systems.

The benefits and value of response systems in active learning are documented, particularly the way in which they engage learners helps to improve satisfaction with the learning experience. They can allow for anonymity, which is useful when a learner is not confident enough to speak out, and they also promote learner participation when they may have otherwise opted out. Advances in technology also renders these systems much more reliable now, with a variety of options available ranging from handheld

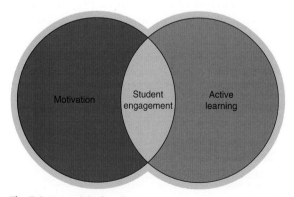

**Fig. 7.2** ■ Model of student engagement. (From Barkley, E.F. 2010. *Student engagement techniques: A handbook for college faculty.* San Francisco: Jossey-Bass.)

clickers to mobile phone technology and other web-enabled devices. Whichever you decide to use, a quick check with your organisation's AV team will help to ease any concerns you have regarding their compatibility with whichever polling system you have access to.

## Learning by Doing While Viewing

Based on our experiences of large group simulation, we have created the anecdotal term of the *Game Show Phenomenon*. This is when members of the audience (in our case, our learners) feel they know the answers to the questions being asked of others when they are simply observing, but they feel less able to respond when the spotlight is on them. Alongside this is usually an element of relief when a question is asked that they would not have known the answer to, or alternatively, an occasional *light-bulb* moment when they suddenly understand a concept they may have previously struggled to grasp. Reime et al. (2017) are clear that observing simulation is a valuable learning exercise for an audience. However, they exert a word of caution as learners still require the opportunity to practise honing their skills and gain confidence in their professional role (Reime et al., 2017). While our learners were unable to demonstrate the manual dexterity required for skills, or the practical impact of human factors, the response system did provide the opportunity to test their knowledge and assess their clinical judgment skills. This was also the first stage for our learners, who subsequently completed a block of simulation sessions. These focused on recognising and managing the deteriorating adult patient, in smaller groups, allowing them to practise skills and to demonstrate their awareness of human factors.

## PLANNING

Early planning is key to the success of any educational activity; however, experience has shown that the complexity associated with large group simulation demands a particularly high level of meticulous and precise planning. There are many potential pitfalls, but these can be overcome if the time is taken to identify each component of the session and to think through the steps in the process. Collaborative working not only promotes a close working relationship between the technical support and education teams but also demonstrates the value of the whole team's contribution. Involving the team also establishes a culture of open and frank discussions, harnessing the concept of a shared mental model (see Chapter 3).

## Education Team Planning

As an educator, you may feel overwhelmed by the amount of planning required to deliver a large group simulation, particularly if this your first experience. Prepare yourself for some pretty sleepless nights too as the preparation gets underway! (Tip: keep a notepad and pen by your bedside, just in case …)

It does, however, get easier, and although detailed planning is always required, the amount of time spent on planning reduces significantly as you and your team become familiar with the systems and processes involved. You will also find that the benefits to the learner make all of the effort required worthwhile, largely confirmed by the palpable enthusiasm from learners during these sessions. The key is to keep your own notes as you work through the stages of planning and delivery, and you should encourage your team to take notes too. This will be a catalyst for the faculty debrief of the session and contribute to future developments. Try to remember that every organisation works slightly differently, and that you will know your own institution best and what works well within that setting. Keeping a record of the experience, including aspects that went well and those you wish to change, will help you and your team develop. Finally, be systematic in your approach. Most things in healthcare now have a structured or systematic approach (e.g., ABCDE approach), and we are familiar with this way of working. Using this type of approach to structure your equipment lists also means that you are less likely to forget something.

### *Example of Checklist*

Another ABC approach:

**A**rea where the simulation will take place (think logistics):
  ■ Will it be compatible with the technology you want to use?
  ■ How will you position the manikin and equipment for everyone to see?

**B**ackground to simulation (scenario writing):
- What are your intended learning objectives (ILOs)?
- Briefing
- Patient trajectory

**C**onsumables (more detail in the next section):
- Airway (to assess and treat from basic to advanced)
- Breathing (to assess and treat from basic to advanced)
- Circulation (to assess, monitor, access, support)
- Disability (to assess, monitor, and treat)
- Exposure (to assess, observe, diagnose, and treat)

**D**ocumentation:
- For the scenario:
  - Charts
  - Profiles
  - Notes
- For the simulation:
  - Briefing
  - Scribing
  - Feedback
  - Debriefing

**E**quipment:
- Manikins
- Cameras
- Medical devices (e.g., monitoring, infusions)
- Consumables

**F**aculty and team members:
- Facilitator/coordinator
- Technicians
- Embedded professional (EP)
- Simulated patient

**G**izmos (technology required):
- WiFi
- Response system
- PC/projector

---

### Time Out: Using the Scenario to Inform Your Checklist

Box 7.1 provides an example of how you can use your scenario and the stages involved in it to develop an equipment checklist. Use this to draw up your own template.

### Scenario Writing for Large Group Simulation

*The secret of getting ahead is getting started.*

*Mark Twain*

While it may seem obvious, it is worth remembering that the first step in planning any scenario-based exercise is writing the scenario (see Chapter 4). Large group simulation can be used to teach a variety of topics from clinical decision making to the application of knowledge of pathophysiology. This means that, before starting out, you need to be clear on the purpose of your planned session and ILOs. With this in mind, it is even possible to use the same scenario for two different sessions. You just need to be clear when specifying the ILOs and amend your scenario storyboard accordingly (see Chapter 4). This is something we have done in the past, where a particular scenario was first presented to explain and teach the pathophysiology of hypovolaemic shock, and when presented again, we focused on developing critical thinking and clinical decision-making skills. This second session therefore focused on recognition of clinical deterioration, delivery of immediate care to the patient, recognising personal clinical limitations, and appropriately escalating care.

It is important to ensure the scenario developed is clinically realistic to promote conceptual fidelity (see Chapter 4). There is a danger educators can lose credibility with learners by presenting unrealistic scenarios which present bizarre vital signs unrepresentative of the patient's presentation. A good piece of advice is to keep it simple. Achieving the balance between presenting an authentic scenario, while still addressing the ILOs, will help you succeed. Remember, your team are a valuable asset, and you should work collaboratively with them during scenario development for large group simulation. For example, the contributions of your technical team can provide an added practical dimension in the form of equipment selection and functionality.

When writing scenarios, we often reflect on situations and patients we have encountered during our own clinical experience. Although anonymised, these reflections enhance the clinical authenticity of scenario development (the previously mentioned

## BOX 7.1
## EXAMPLE OF SCENARIO INFORMING THE EQUIPMENT CHECKLIST

### PRESENTING CASE SBAR*

S: You are working in the Surgical Assessment Unit and are recording the vital signs of a man who has just returned from endoscopy.

B: Mr Brown, a 55-year-old man with a known history of alcohol addiction, admitted with a community-acquired chest infection; since admission, has developed hematemesis and melaena.

A: The patient is drowsy postanaesthetic and there is a gurgling sound from his airway. There is also pink frothy sputum leaking from his mouth. He is cyanosed and has an agonal breathing pattern.

R: You are required to assess his airway and breathing, and to take action in response to your findings.

### LEARNING OUTCOMES

By the end of this session the learner will demonstrate increased confidence, knowledge, and skills in:
- Assessment of the adult patient's airway.
- Recognition of signs of airway compromise and obstruction.
- Basic airway opening manoeuvres.
- Correctly operating suction and oxygen devices and troubleshooting operational problems with these.
- Correctly sizing and inserting an oropharyngeal and nasopharyngeal airway.
- Understanding the complications and contraindications for each airway adjunct.
- Assembling a self-inflating bag-mask, reservoir, and supplementary oxygen device.
- Ventilation using two-person technique.
- Confirming effective ventilation.
- Providing adequate ventilation in an airway training manikin.

### LEARNER ACTIONS AND TRANSITION TRIGGERS OF SCENARIO
- Recognise clinical limitations and call for HELP.
- Airway clearing and opening.
- Oxygen therapy as soon as possible.
- Use of adjuncts (nasal airway).
- Recognise deterioration ABCDE assessment.
- Reassessment and post-incident management.
- SBAR handover.

|   | *Clinical findings* | *Equipment and documentation* |
|---|---|---|
| A | Secretions in mouth<br>▪ Correct use of rigid suction (clears airway)<br>▪ Open airway (head tilt, chin lift) and check patency – Airway clear | Suction machine; suction catheters (rigid and flexible); basic adjuncts; supraglottic airway (with syringe and securing tape); intubation equipment |
| B | Assess breathing and circulation (combined assessment)<br>▪ Respiratory rate = 10, pulse present, SpO$_2$ 79% on air<br>▪ Insert nasal airway, apply high flow oxygen 15 L via trauma mask<br>▪ Sit patient upright<br>▪ Saturations improving, now 92% – still need help...<br>▪ Continuous assessment | Stethoscope<br>Pulse oximeter with probe<br>O$_2$ delivery devices (nasal, variable, high flow)<br>Bag-Valve-Mask<br>Trolley or bed with capacity to sit upright<br>Observation recording chart (e.g., early warning or vital signs chart) |
| C | ▪ Intravenous (IV) cannula in situ (Antecubital fossa)<br>▪ Intravenous infusion (IVI) normal saline (NaCl) 82 mL/h<br>▪ Skin blue, Pulse: 110; Blood Pressure 100/60; Capillary refill time: 4 seconds; not passed urine<br>▪ Attach cardiac monitor – shows sinus tachycardia | Cannula in manikin or ready for simulated patient<br>Blood sample equipment and bottles<br>IV fluids and correct giving set<br>IV infusion pump<br>? moulage for skin colour<br>If available, vital signs monitor<br>Empty catheter bag<br>Cardiac monitor<br>ECG/EKG electrodes |

*Continued*

**BOX 7.1**
**EXAMPLE OF SCENARIO INFORMING THE EQUIPMENT CHECKLIST—cont'd**

| | | |
|---|---|---|
| D | ▪ Drowsy ACVPU Score (Alert, New Confusion, Voice, Pressure, Unresponsive) = **V**<br>▪ Pupils equal and reacting to light (PERL)<br>▪ Keep nasal airway in situ and maintain oxygen at 15 L via trauma mask<br>▪ Continue to observe – ? Glasgow Coma Scale (GCS) | Pen torch<br>Observation recording chart (e.g., early warning or vital signs chart, GCS) |
| E | ▪ Check environment<br>▪ Check medication chart<br>▪ What assessment do you need to make? If learner asks – Temp is 38.2°C.<br>▪ What could be wrong?<br>▪ Complete your SBAR with clear recommendations | Medication prescription chart<br>Observation charts<br>Patient profile/notes<br>Lab results<br>Investigation results (e.g., X-ray) |

*SBAR, Situation, Background, Assessment, Recommendation.

scenario is an example). However, if you do not have a case study from your own practice to use as your canvas for scenario design, you can always call upon a colleague to help, or consult an expert in the field. It is always good to be able to say to learners: 'this scenario presents a real anonymised case study from practice', and by doing so, you can also address the *'that would never happen in real life'* comments from the more cynical learner. Taking this approach means that learners can apply the underpinning science and theory to the presenting case and, consequently, bridge the theory–practice gap. Our experience of large group simulation has shown us that learners see this as a safe way to test their knowledge and gain insight into their strengths, and that they can also identify areas of knowledge deficits they may have in these situations (Simpson and Mackie, 2014). What is important is that your session is evidence-based, and that you demonstrate best practice to learners. Sourcing and applying evidence to inform best practice is an approach that you will ideally encourage learners to adopt.

A key priority is to decide on the trajectory of the patient in the scenario as this will inform the different scenario states. If you are using patient simulators, you must include time to programme the scenario using the associated software packages. Please be aware that programming can take longer than you realise and if you are doing this on your own for the first time, you should enlist help from someone who has used the software before. In some areas, this task may fall to the technologists rather than the simulation educator, in which case you need to be very clear when writing your scenario, especially if a non-clinical colleague will be responsible for programming what is effectively personal thought processes. Once this is completed, you can move onto rehearsing the pre-programmed scenario, in real time. This is an essential step in establishing and correcting any potential pitfalls. It is better to find out in advance when working with the simulation faculty, where issues can be quickly resolved, rather than when in the classroom with learners. We will discuss rehearsal time in more detail, before the main event, later in this chapter.

## Simulation Technical Team Planning

Technical staff are invaluable members of any simulation faculty, and their knowledge and understanding of the functionality and limitations of SBE equipment means they can contribute throughout the whole process, including scenario development.

If using a high-fidelity manikin, your technical team can programme the scenario using the manikin's software package. You must be in close communication and provide clear guidance for them. In our area, not all technical support staff have a clinical background, and we are often guilty of *thinking* we are communicating clearly when, in fact, we frequently use language which is unknown to them. Similarly, the technical team are experts in *their* field, and they also need to be clear when communicating with the teaching team. Working alongside and involving the technical team in the early stages will help forge good working relationships and promote a culture of cohesiveness, where creativity can flourish. In areas where the simulation does not involve high-fidelity manikins, technical staff can contribute in a number of ways including operating medical equipment or filming and recording the simulation for playback purposes.

## Scoping the Location

Large group simulation usually takes place in a classroom or lecture theatre rather than a purpose-built simulation facility. Consequently, to facilitate the effective delivery of the scenario and audience participation, additional aspects must be considered. Both the teaching and technical teams should scope the venue in advance to plan the logistics to help ensure the success of the event. Table 7.1 provides an overview of the logistics which are associated with a large group simulation.

| TABLE 7.1 | |
|---|---|
| **Location Logistics for Large Group Simulation** | |
| Pre-checks required | You must perform your usual checks on manikins and all equipment before transporting. Any problems will be significantly easier to tackle in your own space with your own tools to hand. Re-check all components after transportation as part of the set-up as small cables and pipes can easily become dislodged.<br><br>Decide on the patient's conscious level(s) during the scenario and have an appropriate mode of transport (e.g., a bed, trolley, or chair).<br><br>Consider additional equipment you may require to be transported to the location to support an authentic scenario. This could include a stocked emergency trolley, vital signs recording equipment, dressings, tapes, documentation, etc. (This will have been discussed and planned earlier, and in line with the scenario trajectory, a comprehensive equipment list will have been generated, making this one of the less labour-intensive aspects.) |
| Setting the scene | Consideration needs to be given to the location of the patient at the beginning of the scenario. Ideally, not in sight of all learners from the outset, as this can become a distraction in a lecture theatre environment. You may need to conceal the patient or store this nearby, in which case, you need to consider:<br><br>■ How will you get everything there?<br>■ How long will it take?<br>■ Is there storage nearby you could use temporarily? |
| During the scenario | To engage the audience (learners), they must be able to see and hear the scenario as it unfolds. This is less of a problem in a tiered lecture theatre, as most audience members will have an overall view, but in a classroom or flat seated area, you may need to consider using additional AV equipment.<br><br>In terms of power supply, you need to ensure there are enough and these are both accessible and visible.<br><br>High-fidelity simulators and AV equipment often requires internet access, which may be either hardwire or via Wi-Fi. If you are using a Response System, this will also rely on learners accessing Wi-Fi on their smart phones. Combined, this generates a considerable amount of traffic accessing the systems, and it is therefore important to consider bandwidth, to maintain functionality of equipment and Response Systems.<br><br>When using a wirelessly operated manikin, you should check everything still connects to the system, and identify the optimum position for the mannikin operator where they can have a clear view of events as they unfold and trigger subtle changes in vital signs. If the manikin is tethered (secured), the operator will need to be hidden using screens, or incorporated into the scenario as personnel, but this has the risk of creating confusion of roles and can compromise the immersion for learners. |

### Time Out

Table 7.2 provides an example of the activities required to plan, deliver, and evaluate a large group simulation session. You can use the information given in this table to draw up what you think you will need to organise and who will have responsibility for this. Please remember this is an example, and institution timelines may vary; you need to be realistic according to your own institution's ordering and booking processes.

## BRIEFING

While the core principles of briefing for simulation underpin a large group session, the application of this is quite different to the norm. The following section will contextualise the briefing stage.

### Faculty Briefing and Safety Checklist

This checklist can be used for the rehearsal and the main event; however, it may be that after the rehearsal, you decide to tweak it slightly:

- **Simulation Educator:** Sets ground rules and expectations of faculty members (remember expectations may be different when in front of a live audience).
- **Simulation Technologist:** Provides an overview of any equipment and simulator (if using). Technical glitches can interrupt the flow of the session, compromise the authenticity of the simulation, and consequently disrupt the learning environment.

| TABLE 7.2 | | |
|---|---|---|
| **Example of Faculty Roles and Responsibilities** | | |
| **To Do** | **Responsible** | **Timeframe** |
| Book & confirm venue | Coordinating Educator | 2–3 months pre-session |
| Scope venue | | |
| Book & confirm faculty | Coordinating Educator | 2–3 months pre-session |
| Communicate with faculty | Coordinating Educator | Ongoing |
| Write ILOs and lesson plan | Education Team & Sim Technologist | 3 months pre-session |
| Develop interactive PowerPoint | Presenting Educator & Learning Technologist | 2–3 months pre-session |
| Write scenario | Education & Sim Technologist | 2–3 months pre-session |
| Participant Response System | Presenting Educator & Learning Technologist | 2–3 months pre-session |
| Draw up equipment list | Educator & Sim Technologist | 2–3 months pre-session |
| Book equipment and order consumables | Education & Sim Technologist Team | 2 months pre-session |
| Confirm tech required | Education & Sim Technologist Team | 2–3 months pre-session |
| Book venue for rehearsal | Co-ordinating Educator | 2–3 months pre-session |
| Book scenario equipment for rehearsal | Co-ordinating Educator & Sim Technologist | 2 months pre-session |
| Book Participant Response System for rehearsal | Learning Technologist | 2 months pre-session |
| Develop session online evaluation | Co-ordinating Educator, Learning Technologist & Education & Sim Technologist | 1–2 months pre-session |
| Provide access to session evaluations | Co-ordinating Educator, Learning Technologist & Education & Sim Technologist | On day of session |
| Collate session evaluations | Education Team | Within 1 week of session |
| Feedback course evaluation to faculty | Co-ordinating Educator | Within 1 week of session |

- Communication: Clarify communication strategies between the EP, immersive simulation team, and simulation educator (again, this is different when in front of a live audience, as there is nowhere to hide).
- Support Faculty: You need a back-up plan should technology fail to keep the simulation running. A good strategy is to have a faculty member available to step in, who is conversant with the script and can deliver key information, without the need to refer to paperwork.

### Rehearsal Before the Main Event

The scenario is written, the equipment is in place, the checklists have been reviewed, and we are ready for the simulation. However, before we step out in front of a live audience of learners, there is one final step in the process: Rehearsal! Leaving the rehearsal to the last minute will not allow time for trouble-shooting and can negatively impact on the learning experience. Large group simulations are, by nature, complex, and rehearsal is the key to their successful execution (Ahmed, Hughes and Gardner, 2018). Ideally 1 or 2 days before the main event, the team members should practice the scenario, with the equipment they will be using on the day (*an immersive simulation of the simulation*). This will give the faculty an opportunity to bond and will confirm everyone understands their role, ensuring the team is familiar with operating equipment, and also addressing any potential technical glitches.

This step can create a more relaxed faculty for the main event, serving to enhance authenticity and optimise learner immersion in the experience. While Ahmed et al. (2018) suggest that conducting a final review and practice just before the session is useful, this is not the time for the rehearsal, as the sense of urgency generated by a last-minute rehearsal can be counterproductive. Importantly, learners will sense this, and your message could be lost.

All members of the simulation team should be involved in the rehearsal. If possible, enlist colleagues to be your audience as they can provide feedback to the team on logistics and ergonomics. You need to be sure the audience can see the simulation and should also think about questions learners may ask. If you are using a response system, the rehearsal provides an opportunity to confirm it is working. Deliver the full session from beginning to end in real time, including investigations, examinations, and assessments required as the scenario unfolds. This allows you to work with the team to ensure they are comfortable with the equipment and are aware of the correct responses they must provide. It is also an opportunity for a last-minute check-in with the team, who should be encouraged to ask questions and share any apprehension about their role. From the EP's point of view, this presents an opportunity to confirm and discuss communication strategies, and to establish where they may need to step in to keep the simulation on track.

### Learner Briefing

The pre-simulation brief should clearly outline the ILOs of the session and should indicate to the learners how long the simulation will last. Within the context of a large group simulation there are multiple learners to consider, and their learning needs and roles within the simulation will vary. This can be challenging to manage. For example, our experience of delivering large group simulation has involved a (carefully selected) team of learners delivering care (our emergency team), while we involve the remaining learners (our audience) by using a response system. A response system promotes audience participation and allows them to vote on their understanding of pathophysiology, or the care they feel would be most appropriate. This facilitates active learning, where learners can be challenged and engaged in the decision-making processes. As with any briefing, your expectations, including the role of the learners and simulation team, professionalism, confidentiality, and etiquette must be clarified (Association for Simulated Practice in Healthcare (ASPiH), 2016). This will promote the safe learning environment which SBE is designed to produce.

### DELIVERY

*Learning takes place through the active behaviour of the student: it is what he does that he learns, not what the teacher does.*

**Ralph (1949, p. 63, cited in Biggs and Tang, 2007)**

## Introducing the Scenario

Consider the information to be shared with the learners and how you will achieve this. For those caring for the 'patient', think about communication systems such as SBAR (Situation, Background, Assessment, Recommendation) or RSVP (Reason, Story, Vital Signs, Plan) (Resuscitation Council (UK), 2021), and select one which is both relevant to your discipline and used in practice. A strategy to engage all learners from the outset, regardless of their role in the simulation, is to project the scenario in your presentation for all to see. The ripple theory (Race, 2019) presents seven factors for successful learning, depicting this as ripples on a pond (Fig. 7.3). Race (2019) selected this image rather than a cycle for learning because he considers learning as complex, believing all factors influence each other. He suggests that in order for learning to take place, there must be a *need* or a *want* to learn; this is in keeping with our discussion, earlier in the chapter, of recognising the requirement to learn and motivation to learn as a health and care professional.

Contextualising Race's theory to large group simulation, the scope for initiating the ripples will depend on your location. A lecture theatre with entrances and exits at various points will allow a more dramatic start, whereas a classroom will require some more creativity in the introduction. An example of this could be an audience member (EP) in the classroom

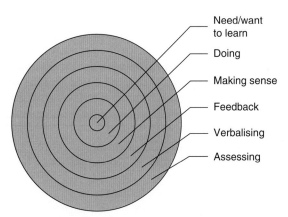

**Fig. 7.3** ■ **Ripple model: Seven factors underpinning successful learning.** (From Race, P. 2019. *The lecturer's toolkit: A practical guide to assessment, learning and teaching*. Milton Park, UK: Routledge.)

suddenly requiring treatment or mid-lecture when emergency services arrive with a patient they have been called to.

## Roles and Responsibilities of Specific Team Members

While the previous section has provided an overview of the process of planning and delivering a large group simulation, the role of team members within this context merits further explanation. Depending on your area, you may have many different team members with specific expertise and experience to offer, which will influence roles and remit. However, for the purpose of this chapter, we will draw upon our own experience of delivering simulation to a large group and provide an overview of the roles and responsibilities of the simulation team involved: coordinator, facilitator, simulation technologist, and embedded professional.

### Coordinator

The coordinator's role is to oversee and lead the event from inception through to completion, and much of the detail provided within this chapter to this point will be led by the coordinator. In summary, their responsibilities can be categorised into three main areas: project, people, and environment.

#### Project

The coordinator will collaborate with the team to lead and oversee the whole project. They will coordinate and involve the team when writing the scenario(s) for planned learning. From this they will organise any equipment required and be responsible for scheduling rehearsals. In our large group simulation, we included an interactive presentation (TurningPoint Polling technology), which the coordinator was responsible for developing and producing.

#### People

Keeping momentum going is crucial to see the project through to fruition, and to achieve this, the coordinator needs to work with the team to set realistic goals and timeframes. This will include bringing the team together and facilitating briefing and debriefing.

The most important people to consider are the learners and, as with all simulation sessions, promoting a safe learning environment is essential. Our large group simulations have taken a number of different approaches, including selecting learners from the audience to play the role of the emergency team, or alternatively, having teaching staff as the team. Bearing in mind the whole point of SBE is to create a safe space for learners, where they are free to make mistakes without consequence, a word of caution should be extended, based on our experiences, when 'selecting' your team from the audience. On the face of it, it appeared that we had selected the team at random from the audience; however, in reality, we knew the students' capabilities, having taught them in class. While the students who were selected to form the simulation team were unaware of the plan in the lecture theatre that day, they were carefully *selected* (and were never late for a lecture again). We must not become complacent and must remember that, depending on the context of the scenario and previous experiences of the learner, realistic, immersive simulation has the potential to evoke an emotional response. For example, selecting a timid student, who could be traumatised by the experience, would not be the desired approach for large group simulation.

### Environment

Consideration needs to be given to the fidelity of the learning environment (see Chapter 4). Within our team, the coordinator took responsibility, on the day, for the fidelity of the physical learning environment, and both the coordinator and facilitator for the conceptual and emotional fidelity. As the coordinator, it is important to be aware that, despite best laid plans and preparation, things can still go wrong (especially with technology). However, do not despair when all goes awry, and the famous song from the film *Chitty Chitty Bang Bang* is a powerful analogy *'from the ashes of disaster, grow the roses of success'*. Our biggest potential large group simulation disaster happened when, due to circumstances out with our control, we were unable to use our wireless high-fidelity simulation manikin for the session. In keeping with the solution-focused ethos

of our team, a member of staff volunteered to be our simulated patient. Feedback from the learners was overwhelmingly positive, a highlight being the 'real' patient. If only they knew! We changed the format as a consequence of this and have never looked back. Since then, our management of the deteriorating patient, large group simulations, have used a staff member as the patient.

### Facilitator

Similar to any simulation exercise, the role of the facilitator within the large group simulation context is to facilitate learning and engage the learners. The facilitator must be familiar with the scenario to take the learner on the simulation journey, as without this, flow can become disrupted. There is nothing more off-putting, or likely to interfere with the authenticity of the session, than a facilitator holding tightly onto a piece of paper and frantically looking at this for cues throughout. While a novice facilitator may feel a level of security having notes to hand, these only serve as a distraction, and do not instil confidence in the learner. This is where a well-rehearsed session and well-briefed EP are invaluable.

As our large group simulation consisted of two concurrent groups of learners – the learners who were immersed in the scenario and the participating audience – the facilitation of learning for each group required different approaches. For the simulation team assessing and responding to the deteriorating patient, learning was facilitated as the scenario evolved. This involved providing clinical information while maintaining a safe learning environment, similar to other simulation exercises described as part of this book. However, in terms of the learning environment for the audience, the facilitator's role was promoting student engagement by way of the response system.

### Simulation Technician

Technological safety should be the responsibility of the simulation technician, and they should be on standby to troubleshoot problems as these arise. Risk of trip hazards for faculty and learners involved in the immersive simulation can be mitigated by adherence to local health and safety policies. In situations where equipment or technology fails, the presence of technical personnel allows the facilitator to continue with the simulation and concentrate on the learning experience.

For the audience to be engaged, they must see clearly what is happening with the patient in the simulation. AV requirements are dependent upon scale, but any environment where the audience members are more than a few metres away is likely to require the patient monitor to be projected to a larger size. The technical team can facilitate this by arranging for a camera view to be projected to a screen to provide a rescuer's eye-view of the patient and interventions in real time (Fig. 7.4). Having a good quality microphone attached to the camera ensures the audience will hear any auditory vital signs or cues in the scenario.

## Embedded Professional

An EP in health and care simulation is a person who is immersed in the simulation, alongside the learner, but given a specific role. They may be acting as another member of the health and care team, or as a relative or carer for the 'patient'. Depending on your area and the scenario, the EP could be the simulation technician, or an experienced healthcare professional (McMaster University, 2020).

In large group simulation, the EP role is key to bridging the gap between learners and the facilitator (Nestel et al., 2014). Within the context of a large lecture environment, where a scenario may be unfolding for the audience to participate, the EP

may offer cues which enhance the fidelity and maintain the immersion of the simulation (e.g., playing the role of another member of staff who can provide additional background information). As both the EP and facilitator are in view of the learner audience throughout the simulation, the ability for communication between the EP and facilitator needs to be more subtle, relying more on body language. Similarly, the EP must be fully cognisant with the scenario (see Top Tips section). Without subtleties in communication and a well-rehearsed EP, the flow of the scenario can be disrupted, which can jeopardise both the learning and authenticity of the simulation.

## Using Response Systems

Previously, response systems required an individual handset for each member of the audience and specialist expensive software packages; however, with advances in technology and smartphones, these are now more accessible and easier to use. If you are new to response systems, the prospect of using them can be quite daunting, but by making time to familiarise yourself and practice with colleagues or faculty members, you will become more confident. When testing the response system, it is a good idea to try to incorporate things going awry to afford you the opportunity to practice troubleshooting on your own. Depending on the size of your group, you may need to enlist some team members to help to troubleshoot technical problems for the audience. If you are fortunate enough to have a helpful colleague who has used the system before, kindly request them to be on standby in case of user error or technical

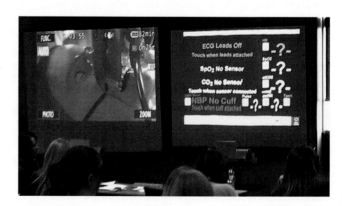

Fig. 7.4 ■ Large group simulation in action.

glitches. Some points for success with response systems include:

1. Always start with a test question, to check both the learners and educators can operate the technology (we used: 'How did you travel today?').
2. Present clear questions. Kay and LeSage (2009) suggest good questions should address a specific learning objective, highlight views of others, expose misconceptions, or generate a wide range of responses.
3. You can generate a sense of urgency by incorporating a timer as a fun and safe way to illustrate how quickly decisions need to be made in dynamic clinical situations. However, be careful not to set too short a timeframe and remember to factor in reading and processing time for the learner.
4. Be mindful of learners who may have additional learning needs and think about how you can facilitate their learning. A reasonable adjustment to support them would be to read the question out while projecting this to the screen.
5. If you are promoting discussion as a way to work through problems, or encouraging learners to explore their knowledge, you may opt to give time out or 'pause for thought'. However, you must strike a balance of time. Too long and the tendency will be for their discussion to wander off, too short and learners may feel rushed. One way around this is to provide clear guidance and a structure for the learners to use.

## CASE STUDY: LARGE GROUP SIMULATION

This case study provides an overview of our experience of planning, designing, delivering, and evaluating simulation to a lecture theatre audience of around 200 undergraduate nursing students. Inspired by recent investment in our simulation equipment, which gave us access to wireless high-fidelity manikins and an AV camera recording system, we wanted to present our learners with an engaging, authentic, and dynamic learning experience. Our plan was to change the usual ABCDE (Airway, Breathing, Circulation, Disability and Exposure) lecture into an interactive session where students could hone their clinical decision-making skills.

To do this, four students from the audience of learners formed the clinical emergency response team, and the remaining learners used a participant response system to vote on the care they would provide. A time restriction was given for responses to highlight the sense of urgency required to make safe and effective clinical decisions in life threatening situations. The software package we used (TurningPoint) allowed audience responses to be recorded, instantly analysed, and displayed within the PowerPoint presentation. From this, facilitators could gauge the level of student knowledge, which informed topic selection for a follow-up teaching session, and students could anonymously establish their existing knowledge and areas requiring revision. When the poll closed, the correct answer was given, and the appropriate care delivered to the patient in the scenario. Regardless of the participant responses, the correct path of treatment was always followed; however, in situations where the majority of answers were incorrect, a short explanation indicating what could have happened to the patient was provided. The rationale for this approach was to present a positive learning environment by demonstrating application of evidence-based practice. For context, it is worth noting that the theoretical material associated with the simulation was not new to the learners and that this simulation was delivered between two other sessions. Before this session, learners had been exploring the structured approach to recognising and preventing deteriorating physiology in critical illness. The purpose of this exercise was to apply these ABCDE principles to a clinical scenario. After this session, students were then given the opportunity to hone their skills in smaller groups.

### Evaluating

While Chapter 9 considers measuring the impact of simulation in more detail, it would be remiss to present a chapter which focuses on a simulation teaching exercise and not mention evaluation. As educators, we

## AIM OF SESSION

To provide learners with the opportunity, through an interactive large group simulation, to gauge their current knowledge and clinical decision-making skills while applying the principles of the ABCDE approach to a deteriorating patient.

## INTENDED LEARNING OBJECTIVES

- Provide learners with an opportunity to develop clinical decision-making and clinical judgement skills.
- Promote active learning and learner engagement within the large lecture theatre environment.
- Present an opportunity for learners to establish their existing knowledge level and recognise any gaps which may exist.

## PRESENTING CASE

Situation (S): You are a newly qualified nurse working in the Emergency Department in a district general hospital. All experienced staff are currently dealing with multiple victims of trauma.

Background (B): A 45-year-old man, unwitnessed collapse. No seizure activity. Loss of consciousness at the scene. No obvious head injury.

Assessment (A): On arrival to the department, seizure activity noted on transfer from ambulance trolley to cubicle.

Recommendation (R): I need you to rapidly assess and manage this clinical emergency!

## LEARNER FEEDBACK

Feedback from learners indicated high levels of satisfaction with the session, and parity in their learning experience. Strengths relating to using response systems included the authenticity of the experience; the opportunity to be active learners while gauging their existing knowledge level; and developing clinical judgement and clinical decision-making skills.

---

should always be striving to improve both our teaching, and the learning, experience. Personal experience has confirmed that it is a worthwhile exercise to allow learners to offer feedback on sessions to establish their level of satisfaction and areas for improvement. Again, based on experience, this is often well received by learners as they feel valued, and it gives them a sense of responsibility and ownership of their learning.

Remember responses are usually honest when anonymity can be guaranteed. Evaluation of these sessions can be approached in a number of ways, and we have tried a few. Taking advantage of the response system is a good strategy to obtain immediate feedback and evaluation. Some systems also allow for qualitative data, and we found this generated higher response rates. We have also used follow-up emails with links to anonymised online evaluation forms and ended the sessions with projected QR codes to take the learner to the online form. However, one fun way was to use social media (in our case Twitter) to gauge reactions to the session. This made for some interesting insights to how the learner was feeling with the surprise arrival of a clinical emergency mid-lecture. The way you decide to evaluate your session will depend on the resources available to you, but it is definitely a worthwhile exercise. We wish you luck on your large group simulation journey.

## LARGE GROUP SIMULATION ON A BUDGET

By their nature, simulation activities are generally expensive to deliver. Factoring in equipment such as wireless high-fidelity manikins, wheeled stretchers (gurney, trolley) to transport your manikin, mobile AV equipment, and clinical consumables is relatively easy for a well-funded simulation centre, but not everyone has access to such specialised equipment. However, with advances in freely available technology, and a little creativity, there is no requirement to be held at the mercy of financial constraints. Table 7.3 provides strategies to deliver a large group, interactive, immersive simulation, and a cost comparison.

| | | **TABLE 7.3** | |
|---|---|---|---|
| | | **Comparison High Budget versus Low Budget** | |
| Item | Cost | Item | Cost |
| High-fidelity manikin | £££££ | Simulated patient (real person/staff member) | Nil |
| Wheeled stretcher | £££ | Table/folding examination couch (your patient can walk to the venue!) | ££ |
| AV recording equipment | £££££ | Smartphone (someone will have one) | Nil |
| IT system to support AV recording equipment | £££££ | Smartphone stand | £ |
| PRS technology | £££ | Online free PRS | Nil |
| Consumables | £ | Scavenged out-of-date consumables | Nil |

## TOP TIPS FOR LARGE GROUP SIMULATION

| Top Tip | Guidance |
|---|---|
| ■ **Journal your experience and make lists to plan for the next time** | Take notes or keep a journal all the way through. Make lists from the beginning which become checklists and templates for the next time. Be systematic and structured in your approach. Using the scenario to structure your equipment lists means you are less likely to forget something. |
| ■ **Start with the scenario** | Write the scenario! Everything else will stem from this. If needed, ask field experts to review your scenario. (Remember: the best scenarios are the real case studies.) |
| ■ **Success comes from good teamwork** | Involve **all** faculty members from the beginning. They will keep you grounded, and realistic in terms of what is achievable. |
| ■ **Order early** | If you need to order equipment, or consumables, do this early. |

| Top Tip | Guidance |
|---|---|
| ■ **Have the intended learning objectives to hand throughout the whole process** | Be clear on what the aims and objectives of your session are and use these to guide the simulation and its development. |
| ■ **Fail to prepare, prepare to fail!** | Always have a 'dress rehearsal' in the area the simulation is taking place. |
| ■ **Think negatively to mitigate for glitches** | Have a plan 'B' ready in case of technical glitches. |
| ■ **Time management is a vital and often overlooked resource** | Be realistic, and if it involves other team members, remember, this might be your priority, but they may have competing deadlines. |
| ■ **Remember the response system** | Perform pre-use checks of devices and be aware that this can be time-consuming. If using handheld clickers rather than mobile phone technology, the battery life in each will need to be checked. Run a test question at the start of the event to minimise operator error (both educator and learner). |

| Top Tip | Guidance |
|---|---|
| ▪ **Embedded professional (EP) is key to maintaining the immersion** | It is a good idea, when in full view of an audience for the simulation, to make small pocket-sized cue cards with vital signs and prompts on. You can go into your pocket for a pen or tape, etc. and have a subtle glance. Also have a copy of the scenario outline in an area unseen by the audience which you can subtly glance at. |

## SUMMARY

With the increasing demand on health and care education programmes, large group, interactive, immersive simulation can present a valuable learning experience. It can be used as a strategy to expose learners to situations they may not commonly encounter in practice and facilitate the application of theory to practice. Although this can be resource intensive in the early stages of planning and delivery, as you become rehearsed at this, it can become an efficient and cost-effective way of guaranteeing parity in the learner experience, and a useful tool when supporting large cohorts of learners. By incorporating the use of response systems, learner engagement can be promoted, allowing them to safely establish their own level of knowledge and areas requiring development. This does not need to be an expensive form of simulation education, and with a little creativity can be achieved on the smallest of budgets with the readily available resources of staff to take the role of your simulated patient and smartphone technologies. Furthermore, with recent advances in technology and a move to online learning, this can be easily adapted for learners studying remotely.

## REFERENCES

Ahmed, R.A., Hughes, P.G., Gardner, A.K., 2018. Simulation scenario rehearsal: The key to successful and effective simulations. BMJ Simulation and Technology Enhanced Learning [Online] 4 (4), 157–158. [viewed 24 July 2021]. Available from: https://www.ncbi.nlm.nih.gov/pmc/articles/PMC8936723/.

Alhoqail, I.A., Badr, F.M., 2010. Objective structured brainstorming questions (OSBQs) in PBL tutorial sessions: Evidence based pilot study. International Journal of Health Sciences 4 (2), 93.

Association for Simulated Practice in Healthcare (ASPiH), 2016. Simulation-based education in healthcare: Standards framework and guidance. ASPiH, Lichfield, Staffs.

Barkley, E.F., 2010. Student engagement techniques: A handbook for college faculty. Jossey-Bass, San Francisco.

Benner, P., 1982. From novice to expert. American Journal of Nursing 82 (3), 402–407.

Biggs, J., Tang, C., 2007. Teaching for quality learning at university. What the students does Maidenhead. Open University Press McGraw-Hill.

Brown, C., Morse, J., Morrison, I., 2016. The integrated use of simulation and voting with personal response systems. The Clinical Teacher 13 (5), 332–336.

Connor, E., 2009. Perceptions and uses of clicker technology. Journal of Electronic Resources in Medical Libraries 19 (1), 19–32 6.

Dufrene, C., Young, A., 2014. Successful debriefing—Best methods to achieve positive learning outcomes: A literature review. Nurse Education Today 3 (34), 372–376.

Durning, S.J., Artino, A.R., 2011. Situativity theory: A perspective on how participants and the environment can interact: AMEE Guide no. 52. Medical Teacher 33 (3), 188–199.

Fry, H., Ketteridge, S., Marshall, S., 2015. A handbook for teaching and learning in higher education: Enhancing academic practice, 4th edn. Routledge Falmer, New York, NY.

Harper, M.G., Bodine, J., Monachino, A., 2021. The effectiveness of simulation use in transition to practice nurse residency programs: a review of literature from 2009 to 2018. Journal for Nurses in Professional Development 37 (6), 329–340.

Hope, A., Garside, J., Prescott, S., 2011. Rethinking theory and practice: Pre-registration student nurses experiences of simulation teaching and learning in the acquisition of clinical skills in preparation for practice. Nurse Education Today 31 (7), 711–715.

Jain, A., Farley, A., 2012. Mobile phone–based audience response system and student engagement in large–group teaching. Economic Papers: A Journal of Applied Economics and Policy 31 (4), 428–439.

Kay, R.H., LeSage, A., 2009. Examining the benefits and challenges of using audience response systems: A review of the literature. Computers & Education 53 (3), 819–827.

Levett-Jones, T., Andersen, P., Reid-Searl, K., Guinea, S., McAllister, M., Lapkin, S., et al., 2015. Tag team simulation: An innovative approach for promoting active engagement of participants and observers during group simulations. Nurse Education in Practice 1 (5), 345–352.

Levett-Jones T, Dwyer T, Reid-Searl K., Heaton L, Flenady T, Applegarth J, Guinea S, Andersen P. 2017. Preparing undergraduate students for the workforce in the context of patient safety through innovative simulation – Facilitator Guide Rockhampton: Central Queensland University.

McMaster University, 2021. High fidelity simulation: Confederates [online]. Available from: https://simulation.mcmaster.ca/confederates.html.

Moyer, S.M., 2016. Large group simulation: Using combined teaching strategies to connect classroom and clinical learning. Teaching and Learning in Nursing 11 (2), 67–73.

Nestel, D., Mobley, B.L., Hunt, E.A., Eppich, W.J., 2014. Confederates in health care simulations: Not as simple as it seems. Clinical Simulation in Nursing 10 (12), 611–616.

Race, P., 2019. The lecturer's toolkit: A practical guide to assessment, learning and teaching. Routledge, Milton Park, UK.

Reime, M.H., Johnsgaard, T., Kvam, F.I., Aarflot, M., Engeberg, J.M., Breivik, M., et al., 2017. Learning by viewing versus learning by doing: A comparative study of observer and participant experiences during an interprofessional simulation training. Journal of Interprofessional Care 31 (1), 51–58.

Resuscitation Council (UK), 2021. The ABCDE approach [online]. Resuscitation Council (UK). [viewed 20 December 2022]. Available from: https://www.resus.org.uk/library/abcde-approach.

Rhodes, M.L., Curran, C., 2005. Use of the human patient simulator to teach clinical judgment skills in a baccalaureate nursing program. CIN: Computers, Informatics, Nursing 23 (5), 256–262.

Rode, J.L., Callihan, M.L., Barnes, B.L., 2016. Assessing the value of large-group simulation in the classroom. Clinical Simulation in Nursing 12 (7), 251–259.

Simpson, E., Mackie, G., 2015. Can an interactive, mass simulation exercise support the development of clinical decision making skills, and facilitate student engagement? In: Jill Rogers Associates, ed. NET (Networking for Education in Healthcare) Conference. Cambridge, England. September 2015.

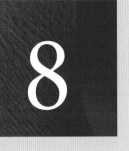

# 8

# MAJOR INCIDENT SIMULATION

CATIE PATON ■ ELIZABETH SIMPSON ■ KEITH
CAMERON ■ STEVEN MORRISON

■ ■ ■ ■ ■ ■ ■ ■ ■ ■ ■ ■ ■ ■ ■ ■ ■

*Successful emergency management relies upon experience and expertise.*
*Leo Bosner*

## CHAPTER OUTLINE

## OBJECTIVES

*This chapter should support the reader to:*

- Discuss the importance and need for major incident simulation.

- Share experiences and provide an overview of the planning required to deliver multiagency and multiple casualty simulation.

- Discuss some of the debriefing strategies used to enhance learning and promote psychological safety in multiagency and multiple casualty simulation.

## KEY TERMS

Major incident

Multi-casualty incident

Disasters and
multi-casualty incidents

## INTRODUCTION

This chapter explores and shares, through a case study, the importance and need for major incident (MI) simulation and the challenges encountered while planning and delivering these events. The stages of planning, the associated risk, the briefing, delivery, and debriefing in the context of MI simulation will also be discussed. Throughout the chapter consideration will be given to all aspects of MI simulation. Each stage will be discussed and, in particular, the importance of debriefing, ensuring this mirrors MIs in reality and to include a hot and cold debrief process following the event. Consideration will be given to the relevant strengths and challenges of an MI simulation when examining a range of theoretical and practical hints and tips.

## BACKGROUND

A definition of an MI was presented by the Joint Emergency Services Interoperability Principles (JESIP) (2022) and the Health and Safety Executive (HSE) (2022). They described this as an incident which is likely to involve serious harm, damage, or disruption to human life, requiring a response beyond the routine. This means any emergency requiring special arrangements which involves input from one or more of the emergency services, National Health Services (NHS), or local authorities (JESIP, 2022) and can be subcategorised as:

1. Initial rescue
2. Treatment or transportation of a large number of casualties
3. Level of involvement, whether directly at the scene, or indirectly at alternative settings
4. Large number of people
5. Need for a large-scale, combined response
6. Activity from the emergency services.

When complex, multi-casualty MIs occur, they require a response from a wide variety of services, and management of these incidents is normally the responsibility of specially trained, highly qualified field experts. MIs, while uncommon in frequency, can be chaotic and stressful for all involved (Hugelius, Edelbring and Blomberg, 2021; Lax and Nesbitt, 2018). Lack of familiarity with the high levels of both technical and non-technical skills required, combined with the low frequency of exposure to these incidents (Hugelius, Edelbring and Blomberg, 2021; Wilkerson et al., 2008) renders skill retention of emergency personnel specific to major incidents a challenge (Larsen, 2018).

Such incidents may overwhelm the available resources through simultaneous dispatch of multiple emergency services to the scene, usually while still trying to maintain a normal service delivery to the public. Similarly, the increased demand for hospital resources may compromise the level of care, and routine care, available to meet the requirements of the general population. Other agencies including local authorities may require additional resources to manage high levels of deaths or provide support for displaced members of a community in cases of environmental disasters.

The risk of acts of terrorism, natural environmental disasters, medical epidemics, or pandemics highlights the need for a robust infrastructure, with appropriately trained response teams and health and care services prepared and ready to respond. Although MIs will initiate the mobilisation of specialist units and highly trained personnel, these do not arrive immediately and therefore are not normally the primary responders in these events. Simulation is the ideal vehicle to prepare those responders who are likely to be first on scene and who will be faced with a chaotic, dynamic situation with little or no immediate support.

A cross-discipline approach is crucial for a coordinated response with effective management of both the scene and casualties (Ashkenazi, Montan and Lennquist, 2020; JESIP, 2022). By allowing practice in the relative safety of a simulated event, learners can develop their knowledge of specific roles and priorities of individual disciplines, while experiencing the partnership working required at such events. While discipline specific training allows individual groups to focus on role specific skills and interventions, training a range of professions together in the context of MI simulation can facilitate collaborative working. Furthermore, a cross-discipline approach develops mutual respect between professions.

## CONTEXT

Disasters and multi-casualty incidents are by definition unpredictable and stressful; therefore, the simulation of these events is invaluable to present learners with an opportunity to practice in a psychologically safe way. Simulation allows the acquisition and development of both technical and non-technical skills required to manage a large-scale incident, while reducing or eliminating the risk to both the simulated casualties and the responders. Being exposed to this type of incident in a safe manner allows the development of confidence, experience, and understanding of the potentially chaotic scene. The use of MI simulations improves and facilitates a shift in the learner's priorities away from the needs of an *individual* patient towards the need to care and manage a *community* within a high-risk situation (Kaplan et al., 2012; Tallach and Brohi, 2021).

There are three main teaching styles for MI response and management: lectures, tabletop, and immersive simulation. The primary aim of the lecture approach is to provide information and signpost learners to clinical and procedural guidelines. This can take the form of either a didactic or informal style and, depending on group size, may include small group discussion as part of a workshop.

Tabletop MI simulations usually bring together several professions, facilitating an opportunity to put into context the overall coordination and management of an MI. Usually tabletop MI simulations are exclusive to those who are likely to be leading and coordinating staff responding to the event. It may involve an exercise in triage, which is the prioritisation of casualties based on clinical assessment. The benefits of tabletop exercises include the low cost and easily reproducible method of triage and developing skills in the management of the overall incident. However, there are some disadvantages to the lecture and tabletop approach as it poses a risk that responders will then be making high-stakes clinical and management decisions for the first time in the stressful and dynamic environment of a real-life MI. It has been suggested that theoretical knowledge is not a measure of clinical ability (Khorram-Manesh et al., 2021); therefore, exposure in the form of complex training including theoretical and experiential learning is required (Hugelis, Edelbring and Blomberg, 2021).

A responder's initial actions when first arriving at the scene of an MI may be counterintuitive, meaning they may attend to casualties immediately, rather than conduct a scene assessment, declare an MI, and communicate with other agencies and field specialists. An advantage of a simulated MI is the benefit of time afforded to learners, where they can process the experience and, through reflection in practice, develop their knowledge. This means they can be more prepared and are less likely to be overwhelmed during a live incident (Wilkinson, Cohen-Hatton and Honey, 2019). Furthermore, gaining experience in the use of clinical and procedural guidelines and checklists during the MI simulation can improve learners' focus. This can provide learners with strategies to manage the range of external stimulus and distractions which are common in the dynamic real-life event. There is evidence that those who have participated in simulation make quicker, more accurate assessments and decisions when comparing performance to novices who have never been exposed to simulation (Klein, 2017). This chapter will draw on our experiences of planning, delivering, and evaluating an immersive, multi-agency MI simulation.

## PLANNING A MAJOR INCIDENT SIMULATION

From experience, we know it takes a substantial length of time and an extraordinary amount of effort, involving all partners, to plan and deliver a large-scale MI simulation. It is easy to become overwhelmed by the prospect, but a strategy which may help is to break down the MI into smaller, more manageable chunks, rather than think of this as one huge event. The first step is deciding the context of the MI, as this will determine the range of specialists required to manage the situation and allow you to establish who you need to enlist as your co-organisers. The context of the MI simulation will also influence the planned learning, in the form of the responders' actions, and having all stakeholders involved at this early stage means intended learning objectives (ILOs) can be developed which will be appropriate for the stage and professional background of everyone involved.

With multiple casualties, comes the need for extensive equipment, and again this can seem quite overwhelming to organise. There are a number of categories of equipment required, and using the A to G approach to equipment lists outlined in Chapter 7 can help guide you (Table 8.1).

| | TABLE 8.1 | |
| --- | --- | --- |
| | **Mapping Equipment Lists to Major Incident Immersive Simulation** | |
| **Aspect** | **Considerations** | **Details** |
| **A**rea | Think about where you plan for the simulation to take place | Logistics<br>Space<br>Safety |
| **B**ackground to simulation | Set the scene<br>Scenario writing | One scenario for every casualty<br>Clear intended learning objectives (ILOs)<br>Patient trajectory<br>Briefing strategy |
| **C**onsumables | For adult and child: Airway (to assess and treat from basic to advanced, with Cervical spine immobilisation)<br>Breathing (to assess and treat from basic to advanced)<br>Circulation (to assess, monitor, access, support)<br>Disability (to assess, monitor and treat)<br>Exposure (to assess and treat) | Personal protective equipment<br>Advanced airway kits<br>Drugs kits, or simulated drugs<br>More detailed account in section on Equipment and Logistics |
| **D**ocumentation | Required for each individual scenario | Triage cards<br>Paediatric triage resources<br>Secure logbooks for commencement of incident log |
| **E**quipment | Be guided by the scenarios (more detail regarding consumables in section on Consumables) | Emergency response bags<br>Defibrillators<br>Medical devices (e.g., monitoring)<br>Trauma management kits<br>Immobilisation or mechanical extrication equipment<br>Traffic Management resources<br>Firefighting or rescue equipment<br>Breathing apparatus<br>Decontamination equipment |
| **F**aculty and team members | Overall coordinator<br>Representation from each discipline<br>Technicians<br>Embedded professionals<br>Simulated patients | Tabards to allow identification of management roles during the incident<br>Senior representation from each discipline<br>Experienced staff from each discipline as facilitators and embedded professionals<br>Technical team<br>Moulage |
| **G**izmos (technology required) | WIFI<br>Communication systems<br>If using cameras permission required from learners and faculty | Response System Communication devices to be utilised<br>Control room facilities<br>Communication centre facilities<br>Body cameras |

### Time Out

Take some time to think about your immersive MI simulation and use the template in Table 8.1 to create a first draft for your MI simulation. Remember, first drafts, by design should not be perfect, they just need to be written, and you can revisit this!

### The Incident

Once the context has been established, it is then time to move attention to developing the simulation around the casualties. Because an MI simulation will involve multiple scenarios taking place concurrently, it is a good idea to decide on how many casualties there will be and draw up an overview of the casualties and their clinical condition as part of the overall plan (Table 8.2). Doing this in the initial stages means you can then focus on writing the scenario for each individual casualty. The scenario writing guidance presented in Chapter 4 can be used when developing the individual scenarios for an MI simulation. However, it is worthwhile enlisting support from a subject matter expert to guide the trajectory of individual scenarios and recommend the order of treatment priorities.

## Time Out

Have a think about the MI simulation you would like to deliver. Use Table 8.2 to consider your ILOs, setting of the scene, the incident course, and an overview of the casualties at the scene.

Once you have completed this, refer to Chapter 4 and use this to develop the individual scenarios for each casualty.

## Fidelity

Fidelity traditionally refers to the level of realism and can be classified as low, medium, or high; this is discussed in detail as part of Chapter 5. Low-fidelity simulation builds knowledge, medium-fidelity builds competence, and high-fidelity builds performance and action Wolters Kluwer (2018). There are three main categories of fidelity within each level: conceptual, physical, and psychological. Conceptual fidelity relates to the authenticity of the simulation, and within the context of a major incident simulation this could relate to a casualty's injuries being consistent with the mechanism of injury. Physical fidelity relates to the extent to which the simulation is representative of the system; within the context of a major incident simulation this could relate to the setting, environment, equipment, and the realism of casualty's moulage (the special effects make-up artistry to mimic injuries). Finally, psychological fidelity is the extent to which the simulation reflects the real situation. While this is powerful and impactful in the development of learning, a risk with high levels of fidelity is

the potential to cause distress to learners. Despite this being a simulation, the realism and learner's response to this can have the same psychological impact as a 'real-life' event (Dias and Neto, 2016) or have the potential to evoke memories of previous traumatic experiences. Therefore, the safe environment philosophy associated with simulation-based education (SBE) is even more paramount. This means a rigorous risk assessment must be conducted to assess the level of risk and strategies designed to mitigate for these. Table 8.3 presents an overview of potential factors relating to fidelity which may compromise the safety of learners and facilitators.

## Risk Assessments

A risk assessment is the process of identifying existing and potential hazards. Within the context of an MI simulation, the risk assessments undertaken will be led by the setting in which the simulation will take place, the nature of the simulation, and the disciplines involved. In our experience each individual specialty and personnel had their own risk assessment tools which were completed, and after assessing the level of risk, a collaborative approach was taken to inform the strategies for mitigation.

The level of risk is usually conducted using a risk matrix tool where a numerical value is allocated to each of two categories: Likelihood and Severity (Table 8.4). Likelihood measures the chances of something happening with the existing controls in place, and severity measures how negative the outcome could be. While a number of variations exist in terms of the number of levels (e.g., $3 \times 3$, $4 \times 4$, or $5 \times 5$), we will use the example of a $3 \times 3$ matrix and apply this to the potential risk to participants associated with fidelity.

Using the equation Severity × Likelihood = Risk will establish the risk assessment rating and, from this, risk can be calculated and categorised as either low, medium, or high (Table 8.5).

Once the category has been decided, a decision needs to be made to determine if this is acceptable, tolerable with mitigation, or unacceptable (Table 8.6).

**TABLE 8.2**

**Major Incident Immersive Simulation Overview**

### Intended Learning Objectives (ILOs)

All Disciplines ILOs:

- Apply the principles of major incident procedures, including:
  - Recognising and declaring a major incident.
  - Understanding the principles of command and control.
  - Demonstrate risk management of the scene.
  - Demonstrate safe and effective triage in association with local and national policies.
- Apply the assessment and clinical skills required in the initial management phase of a major incident.
- Demonstrate ability to respond appropriately to individual casualties, depending on their presenting condition.
- Demonstrate effective communication skills throughout a major incident.
- Demonstrate collaboration as part of the multidisciplinary team when responding to a major incident.
- Analyse the impact of human factors on the quality of care delivered during a major incident.
- Participate in the debriefing process and consider how this informs future practice.

Paramedic Specific ILOs:

- Demonstrate ability to use triage tools for adult and paediatric casualties.
- Demonstrate knowledge in the medical management of a range of casualties with traumatic injuries.
- Demonstrate understanding of the contribution the paramedic role in management of major incidents.

### Clinical Setting and History

Situation (S): Activated to incident.

Background (B): Road Traffic Collison (RTC): Car vs Pedestrians – four-door car with 3 occupants has crashed into a bus stop.

Assessment (A): Multiple casualties on scene, age range from baby to older adult.

Recommendation (R): Your role is to manage this incident safely and effectively in the immediate stages, and work with the multiple agencies involved as they arrive.

### Incident Course

- Dynamic risk assessment (throughout)
- Recognise and declare this is a major incident
- Request more resources
- Triage casualties
- First crew:
  - Incident commander and communication liaison
  - Fire and Rescue Service (FRS) arrive
  - FRS resources deployed to extricate casualties
- Secondary crews Sieve and Sort: Sieve is the primary triage at the scene, using specific parameters, e.g., walking casualties, presence of breathing, or heart rate to categorise casualties. Casualties are then taken to a casualty clearing station and then re-triaged, this is known as sorting (the 'Sort' component).

| Casualty | Presentation |
|----------|--------------|
| 1 | Driver: 30-year-old, conscious, neck pain, crushing chest pain, unwilling to move. |
| 2 | Front passenger: has let themselves out of the car, wandering, confused, and disorientated with obvious contusion to the head. |
| 3 | Rear passenger: 14-year-old, no seatbelt, thrown forward, multiple abrasions, dead at scene. |
| 4 | Elderly lady, shopping trolley: possible fracture (#) pelvis and possible fracture (#) femur. |
| 5 | Child: granddaughter of elderly lady, crying, distressed, thrown 10 meters, compound # humorous, many contusions. |
| 6 | Teenager: school uniform, dead at scene. |
| 7 | Pram: at scene, baby dead. |
| 8 | Pregnant mum of dead baby, abdominal pain, and per vaginal bleeding. |
| 9 | Middle-aged casualty, traumatic amputation of right arm. |
| 10 | Casualty: unconscious, slumped positional airway obstruction. |

### TABLE 8.3
### Impact of Fidelity on Learner Safety

| Fidelity | Factors influencing learner safety |
|---|---|
| Conceptual | Environmental reality may create anxieties regarding safety. <br> Scale of the event: the first responders may feel overwhelmed by the scale and number of casualties within a simulated major incident. |
| Physical | Manikins or actors with highly realistic injuries, through the use of moulage, has the risk of being challenging to the learners. |
| Psychological | Increasing the level of fidelity is associated with increased levels of stress and anxiety among learners. |

### TABLE 8.4
### Levels of Severity and Likelihood

| Category | Numerical value | Level | Definition |
|---|---|---|---|
| Severity | 1 | Negligible | Causing minor injury that requires first aid or less. |
| | 2 | Minor | Causing non-serious injury, illness, or damage that requires medical aid. Not life-threatening. |
| | 3 | Serious | Causing severe injury, serious illness that is disabling or lifelong, or property and equipment damage. |
| Likelihood | 1 | Remote | Unlikely to occur but conceivable. |
| | 2 | Possible | Could occur at some point. |
| | 3 | Probably | Likely to occur eventually. |

### TABLE 8.5
### 3 × 3 Matrix to Calculate Risk Rating

| | | | Severity | | |
|---|---|---|---|---|---|
| | | | Serious | Minor | Negligible |
| | | | 3 | 2 | 1 |
| Likelihood | Probably | 3 | 9 | 6 | 3 |
| | Possible | 2 | 6 | 4 | 2 |
| | Remote | 1 | 3 | 2 | 1 |

### TABLE 8.6
### Categories of Risk

| Low Risk (1–3) | Medium Risk (4–6) | High Risk >6 |
|---|---|---|
| Acceptable | Tolerate with mitigation | Unacceptable |

We have already established that part of the planning for an MI simulation will involve designing strategies to promote a safe learning space. Using the risks identified in Table 8.3 relating to the impact of fidelity on learner safety, we must now apply the principles outlined previously to assess the overall level of risk, and from this develop strategies for mitigation. Table 8.7 provides an example of the next stage which involves specifically identifying risks and planning mitigation for these. It is worth noting risk assessments will be required for the safety of people, equipment, and systems. Therefore, this example is one small aspect of the overall risk assessments required for the MI immersive simulation.

### Time Out

To get you started on risk assessment, take some time to think about one or two potential risks you believe may need to be mitigated for. Use the steps in this section of the chapter to rate the level of risk, identify the level of acceptance or mitigation required and the steps required to mitigate risk. Use the template provided as part of Table 8.8 to guide you.

### Location

It is necessary to scout the planned location for the MI simulation beforehand to establish that the area is a sufficient size to accommodate all aspects of the session. This will include areas for the briefing, the incident, including a space for the casualty clearing station – a breakout area away from the simulation, where learners can retreat to if they become overwhelmed by the experience – and for debriefing. The location should be accessible for both faculty and learners, with consideration given to changing facilities, refreshments, and so on, if required. There must be adequate space and clear access for emergency vehicles, as live vehicles may be required to leave without delay should a real event occur. If using a live location, in public view, it is essential information is widely advertised before and during the simulation. This may include using media outlets and social media to warn the public an MI simulation is taking place and prevent unnecessary panic and calls to the emergency services. All aspects of the location should be subject to an individualised risk assessment (see section on Risk Assessments).

## Equipment and Logistics

In real life, the equipment available in a major incident is limited by the number of responding vehicles and personnel, and it is reasonable to take this into consideration when planning for your immersive MI simulation. Limited resources can mimic the real-life restrictions of equipment during the early stages of a multi-casualty incident, recreating an environment where resources and care must be prioritised. By providing this level of authenticity within the simulation, learners will be safe while gaining first-hand experience of assessing and managing risk, working under pressure, feeling stressed, and experiencing the need to communicate and develop team-working strategies.

### Consumables

Although every responder in our MI simulation carried trauma kits containing all the equipment required, you may find that you are not in the same situation. A good strategy is to approach this one scenario at a time and adopt the principles presented in previous chapters of allowing the scenario to guide your equipment list. An additional feature for equipment requirements for an immersive MI simulation, however, is the importance of collating this information, particularly if the equipment must be ordered before the event. Table 8.9 provides an example of a collated list for clinical equipment and consumables, which may be used by the nursing and paramedic teams attending to casualties at the scene. However, it is worth remembering this is only one equipment list and there may be the need for every discipline involved to do this for specialist and discipline specific equipment.

As providers of SBE there will always be logistical challenges regarding accessibility of equipment and consumables for training, when frontline duties will, and should, always be given priority. A way to overcome this is to build relationships with clinical areas to access out-of-date stock, which can be used in your simulations.

### Cordons and Emergency Vehicle Access

Having the availability of emergency service vehicles and equipment adds to the authenticity of the simulation as this facilitates the practice of establishing the rendezvous point, and scene management, including the inner and outer cordons. Cordons are the method

## TABLE 8.7
### Risk Identification and Mitigation

**Risk Identification**
(List possible risks below and use risk assessment matrix (see Table 8.6) to determine the level of acceptability/mitigation for each risk)

| Possible risks | Severity (Negligible, Minor, Serious) | Likelihood (Remote, Possible, Probably) | Acceptability/mitigation (e.g., acceptable) |
|---|---|---|---|
| **Conceptual** Potential learners may feel overwhelmed by the scale and number of casualties within a simulated major incident. | Medium | Medium | Tolerate with mitigation |
| **Physical** Manikins or actors with highly realistic injuries, through the use of moulage, has the risk of being challenging to the learners. | Medium | Medium | Tolerate with mitigation |
| **Psychological** Increasing the level of fidelity is associated with increased levels of stress and anxiety among learners. | Medium | Medium | Tolerate with mitigation |

**Risk Mitigation**

| Risk | Steps taken to reduce and/or mitigate risks. |
|---|---|
| **Conceptual** Potential learners may feel overwhelmed by the scale and number of casualties within a simulated major incident. | Pre-event education and discussion regarding major incident (MI) management will provide a foundation of knowledge for learners, prior to attending the simulated event. Learners briefed to use phrase 'for real' and would be removed from the simulation to a safe space with support available. |
| **Physical** Manikins or actors with highly realistic injuries, through the use of moulage, has the risk of being challenging to the learners. | Previous teaching around management of injuries using moulage for wounds meant learners were prepared for the realistic injuries encountered in the MI simulation. *Ensure all equipment reflects real practice.* *Actors briefed to be aware of their role in maintaining the safety of learners.* |
| **Psychological** Increasing the level of fidelity is associated with increased levels of stress and anxiety among learners. | Education and awareness of human factors which may be encountered may mean that learners are more prepared for the chaotic nature of such events. Allocated 'breakout' area with refreshments and trained staff available to counsel learners should this be required. |

adopted by scene management personnel to control resources and preserve safety at the site of the incident. The nature of the incident will determine which service is responsible for controlling the inner cordon. For example, if the incident is criminal in nature, the police are likely to take control, or if this is a public safety issue due to fire or explosion, fire and rescue are likely to be responsible. As soon as possible, an immediate cordon is set up before establishing the parameters of the inner cordon and outer cordon. The inner cordon area presents a higher risk and access should be restricted to essential personnel only; however, both services should communicate and liaise throughout, regardless of who has overall responsibility. The outer cordon is designed to protect access for emergency and prevent public access; it is usually controlled by the police, but all emergency services will be briefed on entry and exit protocols. However, it is worth remembering when using 'live' vehicles that these may be called upon to a real event and there will be a need to have a plan B should both the vehicle and operational personnel be called away at short notice.

| TABLE 8.8 |
|---|
| **Risk Identification and Mitigation Template** |

**Risk Identification**
(List possible risks below and use the risk assessment matrix (see Table 8.6) to determine the level of acceptability/mitigation for each risk)

| Possible risks | Level of risk (e.g., low, medium, high) | Likelihood (e.g., low, medium, high) | Acceptability/mitigation (e.g., acceptable) |
|---|---|---|---|
|  |  |  |  |
|  |  |  |  |
|  |  |  |  |

**Risk Mitigation**

| Risk | Steps taken to reduce and/or mitigate risks. |
|---|---|
|  |  |
|  |  |
|  |  |

| TABLE 8.9 |
|---|
| **Collated Clinical Equipment and Consumables** |

| Casualty | Airway | Breathing | Circulation | Disability | Exposure |
|---|---|---|---|---|---|
| Driver: 30-year-old, conscious, neck pain, crushing chest pain, unwilling to move. | A with C (cervical) spine immobilisation Sandbags, collar, tapes, spinal board | Stethoscope Pulse oximetry with probe O$_2$ delivery devices (nasal, variable, high-flow) Oxygen supply | Vital signs monitoring Intravenous (IV) and/or intraosseous (IO) access equipment Crystalloid and colloids fluids fluid giving sets Selection of syringes Cardiac monitor ECG/EKG electrodes Moulage for skin colour | ACVPU = A Alert New confusion Verbal Pressure Unresponsive Pen torch | Personal protective equipment Analgesia Selection of syringes Mechanical extrication equipment Trolley Documentation |
| Front passenger: has let themselves out of the car (self-extrication), wandering, confused, and disorientated with obvious contusion to the head. | Possibly A with C spine immobilisation Sandbags, collar, tapes, spinal board | Stethoscope Pulse oximetry with probe O$_2$ delivery devices (nasal, variable, high-flow) Oxygen supply | Vital signs monitoring Intravenous (IV) fluids and correct giving set Moulage for skin colour If available Cardiac monitor ECG/EKG electrodes | ACVPU = C Alert New confusion Verbal Pressure Unresponsive Pen torch | Dressings |
| Rear passenger: 14-year-old, no seatbelt, thrown forward, multiple abrasions, dead at scene. | Nil | Nil | Nil | Nil | Nil |
| Elderly lady, shopping trolley: possible fracture (#) pelvis and possible fracture (#) femur. | Possibly A with C spine immobilisation Sandbags, collar, tapes, spinal board | Stethoscope Pulse oximetry with probe O$_2$ delivery devices (nasal, variable, high-flow) Oxygen supply | Vital signs monitoring Intravenous (IV) fluids and correct giving set Moulage for skin colour If available Cardiac monitor ECG/EKG electrodes | ACVPU = A Alert New confusion Verbal Pressure Unresponsive Pen torch | Personal protective equipment Analgesia +/− Entonox Limb splints Pelvic splints Dressings |

| | | TABLE 8.9 (Continued) | | | |
|---|---|---|---|---|---|
| | | **Collated Clinical Equipment and Consumables** | | | |
| **Casualty** | **Airway** | **Breathing** | **Circulation** | **Disability** | **Exposure** |
| Child: Granddaughter of elderly lady, crying, distressed, thrown 10 meters, compound # humorous, many contusions. | Possibly A with C spine immobilisation Sandbags, child cervical collar, tapes, spinal board | Stethoscope Pulse oximetry with probe $O_2$ delivery devices (nasal, variable, high-flow) Oxygen supply | Vital signs monitoring Intravenous (IV) and/ or intraosseous (IO) access equipment Crystalloid and colloids fluids fluid giving sets Selection of syringes Cardiac monitor ECG/EKG electrodes Moulage for wounds | ACVPU = A Alert New confusion Verbal Pressure Unresponsive Pen torch | Personal protective equipment Analgesia +/− Entonox Limb splints Pelvic splints Dressings |
| Total Equipment | Sandbags, tapes, spinal board ×4 adult cervical collar ×3, child cervical collar ×1 | Adult stethoscope ×3 Child size stethoscope ×1 Pulse oximetry with adult probe ×3 Pulse oximetry with child probe ×1 Adult $O_2$ delivery devices (nasal, variable, high-flow) ×3 Child $O_2$ delivery devices (nasal, variable, high-flow) ×1 Oxygen supply ×4 | Adult vital signs monitoring ×3 Child vital signs monitoring ×1 Intravenous (IV) and/ or intraosseous (IO) access equipment ×4 crystalloid and colloids fluids fluid giving sets ×4 Selection of syringes ×4 Cardiac monitor ×4 ECG/EKG electrode sets ×4 Moulage ×4 | Pen torch ×4 | Personal protective equipment Analgesia ×4 Entonox ×2 Selection of syringes ×4 Mechanical extrication equipment ×1 Trolley ×4 Adult documentation ×3 Adult limb splints ×1 Child limb splints ×1 Pelvic splint ×1 Selection of dressings |

### Communication Devices and Systems

Communication within and across disciplines during major incidents is essential to the collaboration required for an efficient, coordinated response. Therefore, it is vital to plan for the communication systems and test that these communicate across disciplines before the main event. Similarly, to prevent unfamiliarity with the communication systems and devices detracting from immersion in the simulation, it is a good idea to ensure learners have had an orientation session and opportunity for practice before the main event.

### Mechanical Extrication From Vehicles

The inclusion of mechanical extrication provides an opportunity for fire and rescue crews to practice skills, creating a cognitive challenge which can facilitate learning. The strengths of including a real-time extrication include the time required for interventions, teamwork, leadership, and communication necessary to execute the task which raises awareness of discipline specific roles. However, the associated high risks with extrication mean an interdisciplinary risk assessment must be completed.

| TABLE 8.10 | |
|---|---|
| **Benefits of Moulage** | |
| **Benefit** | **Implication for learner** |
| Enhances the sense of urgency for learners. | Allows the learner to enter and assess the scene and casualties' immediate injuries. Facilitates situational awareness through development of prioritisation skills. |
| Realistic injuries provide a deliberate visual distraction for the learner (ocular glue). | Realistic moulage can highlight the distraction caused by significant injury, which causes deviation from the structured A to E assessment strategy. Provides an opportunity in debriefing to reflect on the importance of the A to E assessment, when presented with a potentially stressful situation and traumatic injuries. |
| Increase of learner's cognitive load and the associated psychological impact. | Increased learner engagement and true immersion in the simulation. Increases levels of stress in a psychologically safe environment. Provide the learner with the cognitive experience and skills to prepare them for real life situations. |
| Participation and application of theory to application of psychomotor skills. | Present learners with the opportunity to practice on what appears to be realistic injuries. Assessment and management of traumatic injuries in a mistake-forgiving environment, bridging the theory–practice gap. |

## Moulage

To promote authenticity of an MI simulation, the application of make-up artistry (moulage) to mimic traumatic injuries is often used within the immersive simulation environment. While moulage can be viewed as a positive element in the delivery of simulation, it historically was considered resource intensive. However, modern make-up techniques, access to free online resources, and a creative faculty team mean access to realistic moulage for symptoms and injuries is easily achieved. A benefit of moulage is the increased realism for the learner which can promote their engagement in the immersive MI simulation (Table 8.10).

## People

Planning an immersive MI simulation requires credible personnel from all services involved to foster a cohesive approach from the outset. This develops a unified team, with a shared appreciation of the complexity involved. Furthermore, representation from each discipline will promote effective facilitation of learning and debriefing. Table 8.11 provides a brief overview of the people involved during the planning and delivery stages of an immersive MI simulation.

## Learners

Historically, immersive MI simulations are delivered by qualified emergency responder teams as part of a preparedness plan. More recently, this strategy for learning has been adopted by undergraduate programmes from professional backgrounds including police, paramedic, emergency medical response teams, and fire and rescue services. Learners within this context may include both undergraduate and qualified personnel, and the opportunity to experience an immersive MI simulation has value for both sets of learners. Undergraduate learners can experience an MI in a safe environment with the support of qualified personnel functioning as the embedded professional (EP). This experience affords qualified personnel the opportunity to participate in a continuing professional development (CPD) activity.

## Time Out

You will have noticed there is a depth of detail required for the planning of an immersive MI simulation, and as with previous chapters, we would advocate devising a checklist to make sure you remember everything. Table 8.12 provides an example of our checklist. Using this as a template for your own event, try to draw up a first draft of your own. This may help you realise that although it is a huge undertaking, by dividing it into its constituent parts, you will see, on paper, that it is achievable (honestly!). Please remember, this is likely to change and does not need to be perfect.

| TABLE 8.11 | |
| --- | --- |
| **Personnel Required to Support an Immersive Major Incident Simulation** | |
| **Faculty member** | **Role in planning and delivering immersive major incident simulation** |
| Lead coordinator | <ul><li>Responsible for overall organisation, including:<ul><li>Making initial contact with stakeholders from all services</li><li>Driving the collaboration between disciplines</li><li>Arranging planning and meetings</li><li>Collaborating with stakeholders to compile plan and timelines</li><li>Arranging and facilitating cross-discipline scenario writing meetings</li><li>Coordinating setting, cross-discipline, and discipline specific intended learning objectives (ILOs)</li><li>Enlisting staff to support as facilitators, embedded professionals, and counsellors</li><li>Leading the cross-discipline faculty</li><li>Explaining programme of events</li><li>Managing flow of learners</li></ul></li></ul> |
| Team leads for each discipline | <ul><li>Be actively involved in the organising group to drive the immersive major incident (MI) simulation plan forward</li><li>Responsible for contributing to setting ILOs which are both discipline and cross-discipline specific</li><li>Negotiating to ensure availability of staff to support as facilitators and embedded professionals on the day of the simulation</li></ul> |
| Team members (as facilitators and embedded professional) | <ul><li>Maintaining the immersion</li><li>Being familiar with the scenarios to provide accurate information when this is requested</li><li>Be supportive to learners and less experienced personnel and promote their psychological safety</li><li>Allowing learners and less experienced personnel the space and time to make decisions</li><li>Act as mentors to support learners and less experienced personnel in their skills acquisition</li><li>During simulation<ul><li>Observing learners – only intervening if safety compromised or lacking skills</li><li>Notetaking to inform debrief</li></ul></li></ul> |
| Debrief team | <ul><li>Leading reflection, hot debrief including evaluation of the experience<ul><li>Inviting learner's reflection on performance</li><li>Return to the ILOs and confirm these have been met</li><li>Take notes to inform cold debrief</li></ul></li></ul> |
| Simulated patients | <ul><li>Follow the structure of their allocated scenario</li><li>Feedback to learners on performance</li></ul> |
| Actors | <ul><li>Additional representation to add to authenticity, acting as members of the public, relatives of the injured arriving on scene, media</li><li>Follow the structure of their allocated scenario</li><li>Feedback to learners on performance</li></ul> |
| Counselling team | <ul><li>Be on standby for participants who become overwhelmed</li><li>Be aware of other agencies to signpost to, should this be required</li></ul> |

| TABLE 8.12 |
|---|
| **Checklist for Immersive Major Incident Simulation** |

### Checklist for Major Incident Simulation

Purpose: To maintain conceptual, physical, and psychological safety of learners and faculty during a major incident (MI) simulated learning environment

| Date | | Venue | |
|---|---|---|---|
| **Faculty/Roles** | | | |
| | Name | Role in simulation session | |
| Lead coordinator for MI simulation | | | |
| Team leads for each discipline | | | |
| Team members for MI simulation | | | |
| Technical team | | | |
| Embedded professional(s) | | | |
| Simulated patients | | | |
| **Housekeeping** | | | |
| Suitable space available to accommodate: | | | |
| ▪ Briefing | | | |
| ▪ Simulation event | | | |
| ▪ Casualty clearing station. | | | |
| ▪ Breakout space for learner support | | | |
| ▪ Debrief | | | |
| Signpost to fire assembly points | | | |
| Toilets | | | |
| Refreshment area | | | |
| Names of professional contacts displayed | | | |
| **Communication/Engagement** | | | |
| Simulation event publicised | | Yes | No |
| Signage displayed | | Yes | No |
| Coordinator and Team leads agree simulation safe to start | | Please sign | |
| Plan scenarios and faculty allocation/roles | | Yes | No |
| Faculty allocated to student breakout area | | Please name | |
| Fire register sign in and out sheet for: Staff Learners | | | |
| Authorising Signature of professional leads to use consumables | | | |
| Authorising Signature of professional leads to use emergency equipment. | | | |
| Social media control in place | | Yes | No |
| **Safety** | | | |
| Adequate faculty available | | | |
| Faculty allocated to student breakout area | | Please name | |
| Professional teams | | Yes | No |
| Simulation faculty including embedded professionals | | Yes | No |
| Technical team | | Yes | No |
| Additional volunteer | | Yes | No |
| Simulated patients | | Yes | No |
| Highlighted at emergency services daily safety brief | | Yes | No |

| TABLE 8.12 (Continued) | |
|---|---|
| **Checklist for Immersive Major Incident Simulation** | |
| Ensure measures in place to maintain safety should the teams be dispatched to a real event:<br>Discussed and agreed with discipline leads<br>Discussed and agreed with simulation faculty | Please detail |
| Inform emergency call centre simulation is taking place in case of bystander making call 999/112 | |
| Audio-Visual Governance | |
| Standard operating procedure for audio-visual recording during simulation is adhered to throughout session | Please sign |
| Informed consent gained from all participants for photography, filming, and audio recording | Please sign |

## CASE STUDY

This section will share our experience of planning and delivering a multi-agency immersive MI simulation. The day began with a refresher of some core skills and an introduction to new skills. These were taught by field experts, providing insight to the competing priorities encountered in practice, and thereby developing a more cohesive approach. Our event incorporated a wide range of undergraduate disciplines from across the university. Nursing, paramedic science, journalism, media, audio technology, and law undergraduates were brought together with experienced fire and rescue crews to respond to, in the first instance, a road traffic collision (RTC) and thereafter a multi-storey house fire.

### PRELEARNING

Learners were asked to complete preparatory work relating to local policies, guidelines, and procedures associated with triage skills. On the day we delivered refresher technical skills workshops to provide an overview and opportunity to practice the skills and procedures required for the major incident (MI) to all disciplines. This served to enhance the immersion in the scenarios later in the day.

### FUNDING

An initial budget discussion led to agreement with colleagues that all disciplines would benefit from being involved in the day, gain new knowledge,

and have the opportunity to practice infrequently used skills and procedures. This approach gained the support of senior personnel and budget holders across the disciplines and organisations, meaning we were able to barter, sharing knowledge in our negotiations relating to costs. Consequently, we were able to deliver our simulation on the smallest of budgets.

### PEOPLE INVOLVED

We took full advantage of the many schools across the university and involved as many as possible, to provide students with a valuable learning experience. Table 8.13 provides an overview of the staff and students involved, the contribution they made, and the learning and benefits to them as a result of participating.

### MAIN EVENT

Our event took a team of three experienced practitioners and academics approximately 9 months from planning to delivery. The steps outlined in the previous section were followed to plan the day, secure a suitable venue, complete the essential risk assessments, and ensure that the logistics were in place. Collectively we developed materials to support learning to meet the ILOs of our undergraduate learners and the organisational objectives of all agencies involved.

*Continued*

## CASE STUDY (Continued)

| Timeline | Task |
|----------|------|
| 9 months | Agreement between organisations/services involved |
| 6 months | Budget agreed/authorised<br>Learning objectives agreed<br>Simulation setting/environment agreed<br>Risk assessments completed<br>Timetabling for any students involved |
| 3 months | Staff availability planning<br>Equipment ordering completed<br>Moulage arranged<br>Proposed timetable for event |
| 1 month | Case studies finalised<br>Patient information and progress sheets finalised |

The simulation was designed to align with the LOs of a university module for an undergraduate Paramedic Science programme. Approximately 40 students were involved in the day, along with 10 media students from the same university. Alongside the students involved in the simulation, there were approximately 20 qualified fire and rescue personnel and 2 fire appliances, 2 qualified paramedic lecturers, and 3 nursing lecturers involved in the delivery of the simulation (Fig. 8.1).

The event was hosted in a fire and rescue training centre and emergency care learners developed the essential core skills required by the JESIP (2023a, 2023b). Experienced fire and rescue and paramedic staff worked as part of the interprofessional team and were taught media communication skills by journalism academics. Journalism students gained experience of reporting major incidents, and conducting press conferences, while law students conducted the post event legal inquiry. Table 8.14 is an example of the programme for the day, which we will refer to throughout the following section.

You will see our event began with multiple skills stations taught by experts in those fields. The purpose of this was to provide an opportunity to practice and review skills before the main events in the afternoon. The first cross-discipline component was based on all aspects of triage, where learners were given the opportunity to discuss their feelings in reaction to the reality of triage in tragic circumstances. It has been widely recognised over many years that triage of a large number of casualties with limited resources can cause anxiety to individuals, even those who are experienced in multi-casualty management. Acknowledging and discussing these reactions allows some level of cognition by the individual should they be involved in incidents such as these in the future (Cortegiani et al., 2016; Sigwalt et al., 2020). The next interprofessional component was extrication from a vehicle, and this was led by the fire and rescue team. This provided an invaluable insight to nursing and paramedic students of the role of these professionals when on scene at such events.

### Time Out

Using Table 8.14 as a template, develop your own draft programme for your immersive MI simulation (remember first drafts do not need to be perfect, they just need to be written!).

### SIMULATED PATIENTS AND ACTORS

For our major incident simulation, we took the decision to divide our cohort into two teams, with each having the opportunity to be responders and simulated patients. A major strength of peers being the simulated patients was their ability to contribute to an informed debrief of learners, while experiencing the event from the perspective of the casualty.

We found that using peers as casualties, while being cost-effective, presented a risk of the simulated patient providing prompts or symptoms earlier than these would have been identified with a full assessment. Because part of the ILOs was to undertake assessment of casualties at the scene, the main objective was for the learner to work through this process, rather than the focus being on a prompt diagnosis. In this respect, 'helping' peers had the potential to interfere with achieving the intended learning, and faculty intervened with a more robust briefing before the second scenario. Lessons were learned for future events.

| | TABLE 8.13 | |
|---|---|---|
| | **People Involved in Immersive Major Incident Simulation** | |
| **Personnel** | **Contribution** | **Learning from participation** |
| Nursing team | ■ Lead negotiator and event coordinator<br>■ Participated in scenario writing<br>■ Agreed organisational objectives<br>■ Counselling team for student support<br>■ Experienced staff were embedded professionals, supporting student learning at the scene<br>■ Supplied consumables<br>■ Simulated patients and relatives of victims<br>■ Maintained safe learning space | **Skills and procedures**<br>■ Triage sieve & sort<br>■ Mechanical extrication<br>■ Spinal boards & airway management<br>■ Immediate management of burns<br>■ Immersive major incident (MI) simulations simulated press briefing<br>■ Simulated press conference<br>■ Provided with media training by journalism lecturers<br>■ Opportunity to be involved in moot fatal accident inquiry (inquest) |
| Fire and Rescue team | ■ Participated in scenario writing<br>■ Agreed organisational objectives<br>■ Provided venue<br>■ Provided vehicle for mechanical extrication<br>■ Facilitated mechanical extrication workshop<br>■ Provided two teams and two appliances<br>■ Provided expert knowledge of scene management<br>■ Maintained safe learning space | **Skills and procedures**<br>■ Triage sieve & sort<br>■ Mechanical extrication<br>■ Spinal boards & airway management<br>■ Immediate management of burns<br>■ Immersive MI simulations<br>■ Simulated press briefing<br>■ Simulated press conference<br>■ Provided with media training by journalism lecturers<br>■ Opportunity to be involved in moot fatal accident inquiry (inquest) |
| Paramedic team | ■ Participated in scenario writing<br>■ Agreed organisational objectives<br>■ Facilitated workshop<br>■ Simulated paramedic response teams<br>■ Experienced staff were embedded professionals, supporting student learning at the scene<br>■ Supplied consumables<br>■ Provided vehicles<br>■ Provided expert knowledge of scene management<br>■ Provided trauma response kits<br>■ Maintained safe learning space | **Skills and procedures**<br>■ Triage sieve & sort<br>■ Mechanical extrication<br>■ Spinal boards & airway management<br>■ Immediate management of burns<br>■ Immersive MI simulations<br>■ Simulated press briefing<br>■ Simulated press conference<br>■ Development of teaching and coaching skills in practice<br>■ Provided with media training by journalism lecturers<br>■ Opportunity to be involved in moot fatal accident inquiry (inquest) |
| Simulation technicians | ■ Advised on appropriate use of technology and manikins<br>■ Technical support on the day<br>■ Moulage team | ■ Working under stress in dynamic situations<br>■ Developed appreciation of academic colleague's experiences and clinical roles |
| Paramedic students | ■ Simulated paramedic response teams<br>■ Simulated patients | **Skills and procedures**<br>■ Triage sieve & sort<br>■ Mechanical extrication<br>■ Spinal boards & airway management<br>■ Immediate management of burns<br>■ Immersive MI simulations<br>■ Simulated press briefing<br>■ Opportunity to be involved in moot fatal accident inquiry (inquest) |

*Continued*

| | TABLE 8.13 (Continued) | |
|---|---|---|
| | **People Involved in Immersive Major Incident Simulation** | |
| **Personnel** | **Contribution** | **Learning from participation** |
| Nursing students | ▪ Simulated retrieval team<br>▪ Simulated patients | ▪ Skills and procedures:<br>▪ Triage sieve & sort<br>▪ Mechanical extrication<br>▪ Spinal boards & airway management<br>▪ Immediate management of burns<br>▪ Immersive MI simulations |
| Journalism students | ▪ Simulated media teams for radio, TV, and newspapers | ▪ Opportunity to be on scene reporting a major incident |
| Media students | ▪ Camera crew, filmed event<br>▪ Obtained footage used in moot fatal accident inquiry<br>▪ Obtained footage to develop reusable learning objects | ▪ Experience of filming transferable to real-world film making<br>▪ Obtained evidence for course portfolio |
| Audio technology students | ▪ Audio crew<br>▪ Obtained audio recording to develop reusable learning objects | ▪ Obtained evidence for course portfolio |
| Law lecturers | ▪ Provided venue for moot court<br>▪ Supported staff development relating to providing evidence | ▪ Opportunity to be involved in moot fatal accident inquiry (inquest) |
| Law students | ▪ Attended moot fatal accident inquiry<br>▪ Provided public gallery and law team for fatal accident inquiry | ▪ Opportunity to be involved in moot fatal accident inquiry (inquest)<br>▪ Practice questioning of witnesses |

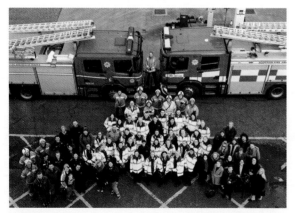

Fig. 8.1 ▪ Immersive major incident simulation team and learners.

## BRIEFING

Briefing for the immersive MI simulation includes briefing for learners, faculty, simulated patients and actors, and EPs.

### Faculty Briefing

To facilitate a cohesive approach, a faculty meeting scheduled at the beginning of the day facilitates the opportunity to set the scene for the day and allocate roles and responsibilities. The faculty meeting presents a team building opportunity where faculty can come together to discuss key points for the day. It is good practice to guide the discussion around both the ILOs and steps to mitigate risk from the risk assessments completed. Unlike other forms of SBE, the faculty briefing for an immersive MI simulation will be co-chaired by the coordinator and representation from senior colleagues from all disciplines. A checklist will ensure no points are missed:

Example of a faculty briefing checklist:

- Welcome and thank you for supporting the session
- Faculty introductions.

| TABLE 8.14 | | |
|---|---|---|
| **Major Incident Simulation Programme of Events** | | |
| **Time** | **Activity** | **Facilitators** |
| 0900–1000 | Lecture<br>Environmental hazards | Paramedic team & SFRS |
| 1000–1200 | Workshops:<br>Triage sieve & sort<br>Extrication<br>Spinal boards & airway management<br>Immediate management of burns | Paramedic team<br>SFRS<br>ENP & Nurse lecturer<br>Burns nurse specialist<br>Simulation coordinator |
| 1200–1215 | Being a simulated patient | |
| 1215–1300 | Lunch & faculty briefing | |
| 1300–1345 | Scenario 1 (Multiple casualty RTC) | |
| 1345–1400 | Scenario 1 Hot Debrief | |
| 1500–1545 | Scenario 2 (Housefire) | |
| 1545–1600 | Scenario 2 Hot Debrief | |
| 1600–1700 | Cold debrief | |
| 2 weeks later | Moot Court Fatal Accident Inquiry | Law Department GCU |

*ENP,* Emergency Nurse Practitioner; *GCU,* Glasgow Caledonian University; *RTC,* road traffic collision; *SFRS,* Scottish Fire and Rescue Service.

- Clarify roles of the faculty:
  - Senior officers
  - Who has control of cordon
  - Embedded professionals acting as mentors to support learners
  - Counselling team
- Explain programme for the day:
  - Walk through the programme timings
  - Inform of refreshments and break times and areas
- Overview of the scene background and scenarios
- Explain the communication system
- Access clinical and triage guidelines
- Session evaluation process for learners and faculty
- Allow questions from faculty
- Final comments

When working with a combination of experienced staff supporting learners in the simulation, there is a risk experienced staff will act as they would in the real world by rapidly processing information and making prompt decisions. In these situations, the learner may be cognitively left behind, still processing information, when the experienced person has already taken action. It is essential all participants gain from the simulation experience, and this needs to be highlighted at the faculty briefing. There are still potentially equal benefits for staff across all levels of experience. For example, a trainee may be able to learn from the experienced staff and develop their decision-making skills with experienced support, while experienced staff can benefit from developing their teaching and coaching skills in practice.

### Learner Briefing

The coordinator should provide a brief overview of the format of the session, which should align to the ILOs. Similar to the interprofessional simulation in Chapter 6, the two components include information relevant to the whole group, followed by information relevant to each individual profession. Recognising that a safe learning space is required for all SBE activities, every effort should be made to achieve and maintain safety within the context of this approach to simulation. However, this can be complex, and multifaceted by the nature of MI simulation. While it is still essential to agree ground rules with learners, the learning partnership will include all agencies involved in the event, rather than just between one professional and group of learners. With this in mind, if working alongside experienced colleagues from multiple agencies, learners need to be made aware of the command structure for the simulation event and be respectful of the rank of colleagues. This respect will ensure that accountability for overseeing the simulation is the responsibility of the most senior officer.

Even though this is a simulated event, the potential risks to all involved are very real and in addition to setting collaborative ground rules, some safety rules will be non-negotiable and enforced by some agencies as a compulsory measure. Similarly, this would be the point to discuss consequences should ground rules not be followed. An example may be that professional conduct is necessary at all times and unprofessional behaviour which compromises safety of any party will result in the person being removed from the simulation.

The briefing is an opportunity to psychologically prepare the learners by supporting and empowering them to make clinical decisions, both individually and within a team setting. If using simulated patients with realistic moulage, learners must be prepared in advance. It is worth being aware that when using simulated patients, these individuals tend to be removed from the simulated scene quicker (Shulz et al., 2014). The simulation brief should be used to discuss the use of simulated patients and encourage the learners to prioritise all casualties, human and manikin, according to their clinical presentation.

It is worthwhile exploring learners' previous experience from practice which may evoke emotions and establish if participating in the simulation is in the learner's best interest. If they do wish to continue, any strategies for supporting them should they require support can also be identified. Within our immersive MI simulation, we engaged the approach advocated by the Fire and Rescue service and adopted the phrase 'for real' as our safe words, which could be used by those immersed in the simulation without compromising the immersions for other participants. Whichever you decide to use, this should be made explicit at the briefing stage.

The checklist in Chapter 6 will work for briefing for an immersive MI simulation, with some slight adaptations:

Example of learner briefing checklist:

- Welcome and housekeeping
- Introductions & creating a safe psychological space
- Brief overview of session
- Focused ILOs for session
- Explanation of hot and cold debriefs
- Signposting for pastoral support
- Emphasise this is a learning opportunity and not a test
- Establish agreed ground rules

Additional considerations for briefing MI simulation:

- Senior officer responsible for safety
- Non-negotiable imposed ground rules
- Orientation to the venue and equipment
- Orientation to communication systems
- The space where simulation and debrief will take place
- The breakout area for support
- The safe word
- Inner and outer cordon
- What will happen in the event of a real incident
- Communication systems

## Simulated Patients and Actors

Simulated patients with realistic moulage play a vital role in providing a true representation of casualties in the simulation, and along with actors representing members of the public or relatives of victims, enhances authenticity. However, being a simulated patient is not an easy task, and these vital faculty members require detailed briefing to promote a safe learning environment. They need to be well-versed in their scenario, and their briefing should include the cues they are expected to give learners, along with details of the timing to share this information. In terms of maintaining psychological safety, both simulated patient and actors should be briefed on observing for signs learners are becoming overwhelmed and need to adapt their behaviour accordingly.

## Embedded Professional

Within the context of the immersive MI simulation, the EP may play a slightly different role. In our simulation, the EP was immersed in the simulation as an experienced professional and adopted a supportive role teaching and coaching skills to learners, allowing them to develop decision making and clinical skills. As essential component of briefing for this group is to ensure they are cognisant of the balance they need to strike to allow learners time to make decisions while still promoting safe and effective practice.

## DELIVERY

There are various services involved in an immersive MI simulation and multiple levels of incident commanders from each discipline, who all have different priorities and responsibilities. All levels of learners can gain experience and confidence which can support their actions during a live incident in the future. To provide a high level of realism, all disciplines involved in a real-world MI should be represented in the simulation event. This requires meticulous planning of staffing and the environmental set-up required, including consideration of communication methods, transportation, and timescales of the trajectory of the immersive MI simulation.

The generic and discipline-specific ILOs of the simulation event require to be clearly articulated from the outset, as context may vary depending on the discipline even in the same immersive MI simulation. For example, senior officers and experienced colleagues from Fire and Rescue, Paramedicine and the Police may focus their ILOs on the scene and logistics, whereas ILOs of trainees from the same disciplines may be more focused on practical and decision-making skills in a dynamic environment.

When using simulated patients, consideration of the environment the simulation exercise is being delivered in requires to be risk assessed to ensure safety of all involved. This is of particular importance where exposure to the elements may place learners and simulated patients at risk. There is a real risk of hypothermia or heat-related complications if the event is being held outdoors, and this risk must be assessed

and mitigated for (see section on Risk Assessments for details on assessing risk).

## Technical Skills and Non-Technical Skills

Learning from immersive MI simulations is best achieved when scenarios allow the development of technical and non-technical skills. Participating in a simulation allows the learner to experience a crisis event, practicing situational awareness and decision-making skills in a stressful environment, with multiple distractions. This enables the learner to build on their previous learning, constructing new knowledge while delivering care in a safe educational space. An example of one priority is triage, a skill that requires understanding. The simulation event provides an opportunity for learners to demonstrate and practice triage skills prior to the mental pressures during an active incident.

### Situational Awareness

When an individual is involved in MIs, a challenge can be maintaining situational awareness (SA) (Busby and Witucki-Brown, 2011; Hunter et al., 2021). SA is referred to as an 'adaptive, externally directed consciousness' (Smith and Hancock, 1995, p. 137; Hunter, Porter and Williams, 2020). When an individual is focussing on interventions when carrying out critical procedures, the potential exists for them to lose situational awareness, by being unaware of their surroundings. For the immersive MI simulation to be useful to all learners and facilitate achievement of the ILOs, a degree of authenticity is required. However, this level of realism is associated with a risk of compromising learner's psychological safety, creating a potential for them to lose situational awareness. This is where having an EP immersed alongside learners can be valuable to support and steer learners should they become overwhelmed by the scene. The EP will be well-briefed on the anticipated ways in which the planned simulation can go wrong and they can adopt alternative strategies to re-engage the learner. If a learner does lose SA during the simulation, facilitated reflection during the initial hot debrief and subsequent cold debrief can provide the vehicle to explore and develop strategies which can be employed during the real-life MI.

## Fidelity

Having a scene that is challenging on an emotional or primal level can create a realistic reaction and engagement with the scenario. While your simulation may have high-fidelity manikins and multiple actors to support the process of patient management, the same challenges can be achieved with lower-fidelity manikins, casualties, and relatives. Consideration can be given to the scene to augment fidelity by playing loud noises, using a low light setting, or adding sensory stimulation – for example, realistic smells. By adding to the authenticity and realism in this way, it is possible to influence performance during the simulation, and also during a real-life event, should they attend an MI in the future.

Any MI can be overwhelming on arrival. Because the immersive MI simulation is a learning experience, we need to support our learners. This may involve considering a timeline by which the scene can unfold gradually, to offer a level of protection for the learner and gradually build on fidelity at the scene. A level of uncertainty can cognitively challenge learners. There is an element of added realism when the true number of casualties is not immediately visible. In our experience we did not present all casualties simultaneously, with casualties arriving from the multi-storey fire as they were rescued, and at the RTC, one vehicle had a child seat, but no child could be found at the scene.

### Time Out

Look at your planning for your own MI simulation and consider your list of casualties. Identify which will be on scene at the beginning and which, if any, will you need to present later in the scenario. Now consider how these will be introduced.

## Cognitive Load

When the learners enter the simulation area, there is always a need for the facilitators to manage information. If too much information is delivered too quickly, there is a risk of losing the level of realism and overloading the cognitive capacity of the learners. This can make them less likely to perform to their normal level and increases the risk of error (Byyny, 2016; Sewell, Santosh and O'Sullivan, 2020).

It is important to bear in mind, while trying to provide a realistic environment for learners, their welfare must never be jeopardised. In situations that require a greater level of control it is important that a safety brief is delivered to all learners, and they understand this by way of verbal confirmation. If acting as a casualty, for instance, during a training scenario with the requirement of being rescued from a 'risk area', it is important that they are provided with personal protective equipment (PPE) for protection. They should be given a 'safe word', which will be mutually agreed and conveyed to all in attendance, which is clear and concise and can be heard by safety officers, facilitators, and learners. This will prompt everyone to cease activity immediately and bring the individual(s) to a safe environment and provide welfare support if required.

## DEBRIEFING

In real world events, debriefing is an essential and robust evaluation technique, used to identify significant factors giving rise to shortcomings or achievements. From an organisational perspective, the process of debriefing facilitates teams' ability to review, evaluate, and amend policies, practices, and procedures (Chouinard, 2020; Elhart, Dotson and Smart, 2019). Within the context of immersive MI simulation, this afforded an opportunity to reflect both from an organisational and individual perspective. For the individual, the debrief after the simulation event presented both the learners and experienced responders with an opportunity to reflect on the experience and return to the ILOs.

### Facilitating the Post-Immersive Major Incident Simulation Debrief

When facilitating immersive MI simulation debriefs, the psychological safety of all involved is paramount, including learners, faculty, actors, and members of each professional discipline. It is important to recognise that individuals react differently to particular incident types. This is based on previous experiences, current stress and resilience levels, personal feelings the incident may evoke, or as a consequence of cumulative exposure to traumatic events over time. With this in mind, learners and faculty are given the option to participate, and if it is established there is a possibility someone's psychological safety may be compromised by taking part, then strategies must be put in place to support them. This may include offering one-to-one support or professional psychological interventions (Raphael and Ursano, 2018).

When undertaking a structured debrief within this context, there needs to be representation from all disciplines involved. As faculty members, some guidelines for this include:

- Co-facilitation (particularly essential with multiagency involvement).
- Confirming who will facilitate the debrief and who will support its delivery. This is usually, the discipline lead for the specific aspect of the incident, for example when debriefing the mechanical extrication, the lead for debrief should be the representative from fire and rescue.
- Because this is a learning opportunity, rather than a real-life MI, it is important to refer back to the ILOs and having a copy to refer to will act as an aide memoir.
- Establish the post-debriefing processes. This may include signposting participants on where to access support, establishing learning and development needs, and action planning to achieve these. This also provides experienced to personnel with an opportunity to draft a final report as part of their ongoing CPD.

As with all debriefing activities in simulation, the facilitator must work with the learners and co-faculty to generate ground rules. While the standard rules of debriefing apply, to maintain participant's psychological safety, some additional aspects to consider following immersive MI simulation include:

- Involve all who were directly involved and those observing. For example, when discussing mechanical extrication, we included the paramedic and fire and rescue teams directly involved in the extrication itself, and colleagues, who, as observers, were able to offer valuable contributions to the discussion.
- The debrief should be facilitated with transparency and a supportive learning environment, where learners feel valued and safe to contribute.
- Learners need to be respectful of each other, and the command-and-control structure of all contributing disciplines, as this is essential to decision making processes and accountability.

It is good practice to mirror real-world debriefing strategies used by the emergency services within the context of an immersive MI simulation. This adds to the authenticity of the experience while also promoting psychological safety for all involved. Debriefing within this context takes part in two stages: the hot debrief (at the scene) and the cold debrief (usually a minimum of 24 hours after the event). Information from the hot debrief informs the agenda for the cold debrief.

## Hot Debrief

The hot debrief should take place at the scene immediately after the incident. It must include all disciplines involved in the response, with the purpose of reviewing activity at the scene and presenting an opportunity for shared learning, while promoting collaborative working (Brazil and Williams, 2021). A hot debrief is considered mandatory when responding to MI events in the real world (Watkins et al., 2019). Therefore, by including this in the simulation exercise, learners will have an opportunity to practice, develop situational awareness, and appreciate the benefits of the process.

The immediacy of feedback from a credible and knowledgeable facilitator will help learners achieve valuable experience through reflection. This will serve to develop the learner's awareness of the intrinsic and extrinsic factors which may influence their actions in future incidents of this type (Hunter et al., 2021; Luiijf and Klaver, 2009). The role of the debriefer during a hot debrief is to facilitate the session effectively and safely. There are several tools for hot debriefing available; they follow a structure of rapid review of a situation, and an example of this is the 'TAKE STOCK' Hot debrief tool (Sugarman et al., 2021):

Take an instruction sheet.
Ask "Is everyone OK?"
Know if anyone needs a break.
Equipment issues?
Summarise the event.
Things that went well.
Opportunities to learn.

Cold debrief necessary?

Know who is present.

Although the TAKE STOCK acronym was originally designed for use in the emergency department, it is transferable to the immersive MI simulation, with the caveat that as a learning experience, it is essential facilitators include the ILOs as part of the framework for discussion. From our experience, these included:

- Team performance
- Procedures employed and their effectiveness
- Hazard and risk identification
- How effective were the control measures (cordons)
- Organisational learning in relation to policies, procedures, health and safety, equipment, vehicles, partner agency working

## Cold Debrief

This structured debrief is informed by the information gained at the hot debrief stage. The preparation for a cold debrief involves collating details of the event from the outset, including timelines, disciplines involved, and the sequence of actions throughout the event (Salik and Paige, 2020), in our case an immersive MI simulation. In real life, the cold debrief should be conducted as soon as practical after the event, to ensure accuracy of information from those involved (Argintaru et al., 2020). However, in a simulated MI simulation, you may be constrained by the availability of learners and faculty and therefore, this may need to be conducted sooner, potentially immediately after the hot debrief. Within the context of the cold debrief, the use of appropriate humour and ensuring a level of credibility is instrumental in making the learner feel that they are not alone. To promote a culture of safety and a collegiate approach, using language like we, us, our, and so on promotes the concept of being part of a team.

To support a learning culture, it is vitally important that individuals can raise learning points, have a process for them to be progressed and to receive feedback as to whether the point(s) raised have been actioned or otherwise. A key component of any debrief process is the ability to progress identified learning points raised by learners, and support may be required to help them action plan for their learning.

## TOP TIPS FOR IMMERSIVE MAJOR INCIDENT SIMULATION

| Top Tip | Guidance |
| --- | --- |
| - Plan, Plan, Plan | Make lists and have lists of lists. |
| | Involve your stakeholders from the outset and keep them involved. |
| | Meet with seniors and budget holders early in the process and confirm buy in. |
| | Get a realistic timeline drawn up. |
| | Have regular meetings and an action for each (e.g., scenario writing sessions). |
| | Get equipment lists drawn up early and start collecting. |
| - Someone needs to be in control and have oversight | Allocate the main coordinator and plan meetings in advance. |
| | Set up ground rules with the organising team. |
| | If someone cannot be represented at a meeting, ask for an alternative representative. |
| | Keep the momentum going. |
| - Budget | Find out if you need funding or if you could barter services. |
| | Collect out-of-date equipment. |
| - Safety first! | Risk assess each step of the way and plan the strategies to mitigate for any risk. |
| - Teamwork makes a dream work | Build good relationships with all stakeholders. |
| | Enlist your team early on to have commitment. |
| | Slightly over recruit in case of last-minute call-offs. |

| Top Tip | Guidance |
|---|---|
| ■ **Do not forget the moulage** | Allocate the role and again, draw up a list of requirements for realistic moulage according to the mechanism of injuries of the casualties. |

## SUMMARY

Not all MI simulations need to be immersive, and it should be acknowledged different approaches have strengths depending on the ILOs. For example, 'tabletop' exercises are ideal for developing skills around scene management needs, and paper triage experiences allow the processing of guidelines and algorithms. However, a major strength of an immersive MI simulation is the opportunity afforded to all participants to experience a chaotic, unpredictable, dynamic environment where learners can gain experience and build confidence. There are many considerations to include when planning these simulated events such as the level of fidelity, learner experience, and equipment required. While debriefing is an essential component for all SBE activities, the role the two stages of debrief (hot and cold) plays in psychological safety is even more paramount within the context of immersive MI simulation.

## REFERENCES

Argintaru, N., Li, W., Hicks, C., White, K., McGowan, M., Gray, S., Petrosoniak, A., 2021. An active shooter in your hospital: a novel method to develop a response policy using in situ simulation and video framework analysis. Disaster Medicine and Public Health Preparedness 15 (2), 223–231. https://doi.org/10.1017/dmp.2019.161.

Ashkenazi, I., Montán, K.L., Lennquist, S., 2020. Mass casualties incident: Education, simulation, and training. In: WSES Handbook of Mass Casualties Incidents Management. Springer, Cham, pp. 167–175.

Brazil, V., Williams, J., 2021. How to lead a hot debrief in the emergency department. EMA-Emergency Medicine Australasia 33 (5), 925–927.

Busby, S., Witucki-Brown, J., 2011. Theory development for situational awareness in multi-casualty incidents. Journal of emergency nursing 37 (5), 444–452.

Byyny, R.L., 2016 Autumn. 2016. Information and cognitive overload: How much is too much? The Pharos of Alpha Omega Alpha-Honor Medical Society 79 (4), 2–7. PMID: 29481015.

Chouinard, J., 2020. Paramedics and The Chance of a Better Outcome: Psychological Health and Safety and Employer Liability. University of Saskatchewan, Saskatchewan, Canada.

Cortegiani, A., Russotto, V., Gregoretti, C., Giarratano, A., Antonelli, M., 2016. Medical simulation for ICU staff: Does it influence safety of care? Intensive Care Medicine 42 (4) 635–635.

Dias, R.D., Neto, A.S., 2016. Stress levels during emergency care: A comparison between reality and simulated scenarios. Journal of critical care, 33, pp.8-13.

Elhart, M.A., Dotson, J., Smart, D., 2019. Psychological debriefing of hospital emergency personnel: review of critical incident stress debriefing. International Journal of Nursing Student Scholarship 6.

Health and Safety Executive, 2022. Investigation - Stage 1: Receive incident details - Additional guidance. [online]. Available from https://www.hse.gov.uk/foi/internalops/og/ogprocedures/investigation/majorincident.htm#:~:text=Definition%20of%20major%20incident,establishment%20or%20transient%20work%20activity.

Hugelius, K., Edelbring, S., Blomberg, K., 2021. Prehospital major incident management: How do training and real-life situations relate? A qualitative study. BMJ Open 11 (9), e048792.

Hunter, J., Porter, M., Phillips, A., Evans-Brave, M., Williams, B., 2021. Do paramedic students have situational awareness during high-fidelity simulation? A mixed-methods pilot study. International Emergency Nursing 56, 100983.

Hunter, J., Porter, M., Williams, B., 2020. Towards a theoretical framework for situational awareness in paramedicine. Safety Science 122, 104528.

Joint Emergency Services Interoperability Principles, 2022. Major Incident.

Joint Emergency Services Interoperability Principles (JESIP), 2023a. Early Stages of an Incident & M/ETHANE [online]. JESIP. Available from: https://jesip.org.uk/early-stages-methane.

Joint Emergency Services Interoperability Principles (JESIP), 2023b. The Five Principles [online]. JESIP. Available from: https://jesip.org.uk/five-principles.

Kaplan, B.G., Connor, A., Ferranti, E.P., Holmes, L., Spencer, L., 2012. Use of an emergency preparedness disaster simulation with undergraduate nursing students. Public Health Nursing 29 (1), 44–51.

Khorram-Manesh, A., Goniewicz, K., Hertelendy, A., Dulebenets, M. (Eds.), 2021. Handbook of Disaster and Emergency Management. Kompendiet, Sweden.

Klein, G., 2017. Sources of Power: How People Make Decisions. MIT Press, Cambridge, MA.

Larsen, D.P., 2018. Planning education for long-term retention: The cognitive science and implementation of retrieval practice. In Seminars in Neurology 38 (04), 449–456. Thieme Medical Publishers.

Lax, P., Nesbitt, I., 2018. Major incidents: An overview. Surgery (Oxford) 36 (8), 386–388.

Luiijf, E., Klaver, M., 2009. Insufficient situational awareness about critical infrastructures by emergency management. C3I for Crisis, Emergency and Consequence Management May. pp 10/11-10/10.

Raphael, B., Ursano, R.J., 2018. Psychological debriefing. In: Sharing the Front Line and the Back Hills. Routledge, Milton Park, UK, pp. 343–352.

Salik, I., Paige, J.T., 2020. Debriefing the interprofessional team in medical simulation. In: StatPearls [Internet]. StatPearls Publishing, Treasure Island FL. 2023 Jan. PMID: 32119413.

Sewell, J.L., Santhosh, L., O'Sullivan, P.S., 2020. How do attending physicians describe cognitive overload among their workplace learners? Medical Education 54 (12), 1129–1136.

Sigwalt, F., Petit, G., Evain, J.N., Claverie, D., Bui, M., Guinet-Lebreton, A., et al., 2020. Stress management training improves overall performance during critical simulated situations: A prospective randomized controlled trial. Anesthesiology 133 (1), 198–211.

Smith, K., Hancock, P.A., 1995. Situation awareness is adaptive, externally directed consciousness. Human Factors 37 (1), 137–148.

Sugarman, M., Graham, B., Langston, S., Nelmes, P., Matthews, J., 2021. Implementation of the 'TAKE STOCK' Hot Debrief Tool in the ED: A quality improvement project. Emergency Medicine Journal 38 (8), 579–584.

Tallach, R., Brohi, K., 2021. Embracing uncertainty in mass casualty incidents. British Journal of Anaesthesia.

Watkins, N., Johnston, A.N., McNamee, P., Muter, N., Huang, C., Ling Li, Y., et al., 2019. Preparing for mass casualties: Improving staff preparedness and hospital operations through multidisciplinary simulation training in disaster management. Prehospital and Disaster Medicine 34 (s1), s81–s82.

Wilkerson, W., Avstreih, D., Gruppen, L., Beier, K.P., Woolliscroft, J., 2008. Using immersive simulation for training first responders for mass casualty incidents. Academic Emergency Medicine 15 (11), 1152–1159.

Wilkinson, B., Cohen-Hatton, S.R., Honey, R.C., 2019. Decision-making in multi-agency groups at simulated major incident emergencies: in situ analysis of adherence to UK doctrine. Journal of Contingencies and Crisis Management 27 (4), 306–316.

Wolters Kluwer 2018. Increasing fidelity and realism in simulation for nursing students. [online] Available at: https://www.wolterskluwer.com/en/expert-insights/increasing-fidelity-and-realism-in-simulation. Accessed 3rd July 2023.

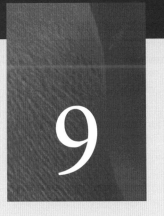

# 9

# MEASURING THE IMPACT OF SIMULATION-BASED EDUCATION

JERRY MORSE ■ ANDREA BAKER ■ CLAIRE McGUINNESS

## CHAPTER OUTLINE

## OBJECTIVES

*This chapter should support the reader to:*

■ Develop an understanding of simulation-based education (SBE) evaluation and research.

■ Consider the role and importance of evaluation and research to improve the quality of SBE activities and health and care delivery.

■ Consider the rationale, planning, and application of both SBE evaluation and research projects, and in what context to apply each.

■ Recognise the importance of measuring and understanding the impact of SBE on learners' practice and health and care delivery.

## INTRODUCTION

This book has focused on guiding and supporting the reader to achieve a better understanding of simulation-based education (SBE), and activities which can be planned and delivered as part of this. However, evaluation and, in some cases research, are of equal importance because these facilitate a better understanding of what has been successful and what improvements are required. For those responsible for measuring output from the delivery of their SBE activities, this chapter will provide guidance and strategies for audit and measurement of impact. Examples of tools that can be used to generate and provide data on the impact of SBE on both practice and learners' experience will also be shared.

## KEY TERMS

| | |
|---|---|
| Simulation-based education | Research |
| Quality improvement | Data collection |
| Inter-professional | Tools |
| Uni-professional | Impact |
| Evaluation | Educator |
| | Facilitator |

## BACKGROUND

*In a constrained economic climate, where simulation education is expanding, planners and managers need assurance that simulation is cost effective, evidence based and led by prepared trainers. Evaluations that address students/trainees' experience, learning, behaviours and the subsequent impact on resources and patient outcomes will become increasingly important.*

*Gobbi et al., 2012, p. 412*

As an educator or facilitator of SBE, there is a responsibility to measure the impact of any learning activities and the learners' experience of these. As part of this, there is also a responsibility to undertake measures to promote quality improvement going forward.

In recent years it is notable that SBE research and evaluation has grown, and evaluation in particular is now an integral part of the delivery of SBE, irrespective of the learning environment. However, to be considered as an effective learning technique, SBE must also be measured in terms of its indirect effect on patient outcomes and patient safety.

Historically, the aviation industry has always recognised the benefits of SBE. Because of this, when asked to explain the impact of SBE on practice and patient outcomes, it is possible to draw on the example of Captain Chesley Sullenberger, the pilot who had to make an emergency landing on the Hudson River, New York, in 2009. Using the animated reconstruction of the flight, including the 2 minutes and 38 seconds from take-off to landing, and listening to the voice recording of the conversation between the pilots and flight control, it is possible to explore the technical and non-technical aspects which ensued in that very short timeframe, and how the crew were able to avert a disaster.

When considering this event, while the pilot had not practiced an emergency landing on the Hudson River, perhaps the key to the safe landing lies in the fact that all pilots must undergo simulation training as part of safety measures in the aviation industry. Furthermore, while landing on water was a consequence of the skill of the pilots, that was only the beginning of the presenting situation. Passengers then had to be evacuated from the aeroplane before it sank. This was the remit of the cabin crew who,

once again, had practiced this scenario in simulation. Therefore, when reviewing this real-life emergency, the importance of incorporating simulation as a training and education modality is clear, particularly in terms of safe landing, evacuation, and overall preservation of life for those involved. Similarly, when listening to the voice recordings of this landing, it is possible to analyse the non-technical skills, in particular communication between the pilots and the flight controllers, which enabled the generation of multiple options for an emergency landing. Overall, the rehearsal of both technical and non-technical skills in this case helped to ensure no loss of life and passenger and crew safety.

The complete event highlights how both technical and non-technical skills can be honed through the use of simulation. While, in this example, simulated practice took place separately for each group, interprofessional working was key, as was the focus on knowledge, skills and, human factors, including rehearsing for events which it was hoped would never take place (Abildgren et al., 2022). This is important as close comparisons can be drawn between the goals of simulation in aviation and the goals when delivering SBE in health and care. Examples of this are evident in undergraduate health and care education where students from various professions utilise simulation in some form or another to assist in meeting the learning outcomes (LOs) required for programme completion. While this is more often than not performed uniprofessionally, the evidence continues to grow for an interprofessional approach in simulation (refer to Chapter 6), with those from different health and care professions learning together in teams as they would in practice. The challenge is therefore to measure the impact of both uniprofessional and interprofessional SBE.

## CONTEXT

The concept of measuring the output and the effect on learners' practice and care delivery outcomes may be daunting. It may also be daunting to embark on an evaluation of faculty's experience of SBE delivery. However, this chapter will focus on debunking the myths which perhaps surround the creation and implementation of robust evaluation and quality improvement. Research, in the context of SBE, will also be touched upon to present a complete overview of the possibilities when measuring impact and planning improvements in SBE.

Irrespective of whether or not SBE evaluation or research is chosen, it is important to acknowledge that ethical approval will always be required when conducting research and, in some circumstances, may also be required for evaluation. Either way, all research and/or evaluation must be developed with the underpinning mantra that ethical principles will be followed to protect the safety and rights of those supporting your inquiry (University of Cambridge Teaching Centre for Teaching and Learning, 2023). It is good practice to seek the advice of your local, or if necessary, regional, research ethics committee and record their response. It is also important to recognise that you may need proof of ethics advice if wishing to publish or present.

Before considering context, it is helpful to compare evaluation and research in practical terms. Mathieson (2007) explored this comparison in general terms, and this work has now been applied in the context of SBE (Table 9.1).

It is also important to consider whether or not ethical approval is likely to be required. For research, the answer to this question will always be yes; however, for evaluation, the answer requires more thought. Focusing on evaluation, it is important to be clear about the context of the evaluation, including the purpose, data to be gathered, potential impact on respondents, and what the data collected will be used for. These considerations are pivotal when determining whether or not ethical approval will be required.

Twycross and Shorten (2014, p. 65) consider research, audit, and service evaluation in the context of health and care, exploring the similarities and differences of each. They are clear that, in some cases, ethical approval may not be required for evaluation, stating *Service evaluation seeks to assess how well a service is achieving its intended aims. It is undertaken to benefit the people using a particular healthcare service and is designed and conducted with the sole purpose of defining or judging the current service. The results of service evaluations are mostly used to generate information that can be used to inform local decision-making'.* Although this explanation is provided in the context of healthcare, it is arguable that this can be transferred to the health and care SBE environment, providing guidance around how best to approach evaluation if there are no plans to seek ethical approval. The similarities are clear in that, often, evaluation of SBE focuses on consideration of what worked well, and how best to improve SBE activities moving forward. However, it is important to be aware that, if there is intention to publish/disseminate evaluation findings more widely, ethical approval will most likely be required, emphasising again the importance of being clear regarding the context within which the evaluation will take place.

Irrespective of this, and whether or not you choose to embark on evaluation or research, the primary concern must also be focused on those who are willing to share information with you regarding their engagement with SBE. Participation must always be based on the premise of choice and anonymity, and confidentiality should be protected. If seeking information from students, it must be clear that there will be no repercussions should they decide not to take part, or should their feedback be negative. Adopting this stance at the outset will help to ensure a safe environment for the provision of feedback on engagement.

## TABLE 9.1
### Comparison of Key Characteristics of Evaluation and Research

| Evaluation | Research |
|---|---|
| Evaluation can focus on particular aspects of the situation-based education (SBE) to learn more | Research can focus on the SBE activity overall and can provide more generalisable and/or transferable conclusions |
| Evaluation can be designed to support improvement in SBE | Research can be designed to prove that an aspect of SBE, or SBE activity, works well |
| Evaluation can provide the basis for decision-making when creating SBE activities or interventions | Research can provide the basis to reach conclusions and, where appropriate, to identify further areas for research |
| Evaluation can examine how well an SBE intervention or activity works (delivery) | Research can help to determine how the SBE activity or intervention works (process) |
| Evaluation can determine what is valuable about an SBE activity | Research can determine what the SBE activity is in more depth |

Overall, the best advice is to seek the guidance of your local research ethics committee before embarking on any SBE research or evaluation. This will help to ensure that you follow the correct process from the outset and will also help to avoid any ethical complications as your project progresses.

## MEASURING THE IMPACT OF SIMULATION-BASED EDUCATION

Before considering how best to ascertain impact and learn about experience, it is important to understand that the impact on and experience of patients, whilst stemming from the SBE activity, will be indirect and therefore more challenging to measure and quantify. However, it is possible to measure a number of SBE variables, depending on the focus of your interest and intelligence gathering. From an evaluation and research perspective, this could include the (not an exhaustive list):

- Learners' experience of the SBE activity generally
- Impact on learners' skill development
- Impact on learners' knowledge
- Impact on learners' competence (including application to practice)
- Impact on learners' confidence
- Faculty's experience of SBE participation

Moving forward, this chapter will now present strategies and tools which can be applied to enable evaluation and/or research for quality improvement.

## SIMULATION-BASED EDUCATION AND EVALUATION

It has already been acknowledged that SBE has an established role in the education and training of health and care professionals. However, its function as a health and care quality improvement (QI) tool remains relatively unknown and continues to evolve (Buljac-Samardizic et al, 2020). As educators, there is a need to continue adding to the evidence base of SBE, and its impact, to understand what is effective and the potential indirect effect on care delivery outcomes. Whether this is from improved interprofessional team working, improved care targets, or to test new facilities prior to commissioning, the SBE undertaken can provide the data to support evaluation and understand

the impact educational modality. This may then lead to the planning and initiation of research to explore in more depth.

### Rationale for Evaluation

At the outset of this chapter, the options of evaluation or research were introduced. Before embarking on either, it is important to understand the reasons which underpin the desire to gather information. This will ensure that the information gathering process is suitably informed and that the data collected will serve the desired purpose.

Considering evaluation, the rationale is often multifaceted and can be founded in a desire to understand learner or faculty experience of SBE in greater depth. This narrative, if detailed, can enable a greater understanding of the learners' experience, as well as providing some insight into changes in confidence and/or competence levels as a result of engaging with SBE (Sterner, Skyvell Nilsson and Eklund, 2023). From the perspective of faculty, the evaluation process will most likely focus on their experience of developing and delivering SBE. Gaining this insight will enable ongoing quality improvement of all aspects of the SBE process.

Considering both learners and faculty together, the key rationale for evaluation relates to the real-time nature of the intelligence which can be gathered, as well as the speed with which this information can be acted upon. An added benefit to evaluation relates to the timing of the process. In most circumstances evaluation will take place immediately pre and/or post-simulation activity. Again, in terms of rationale, this is important as ongoing SBE evaluation enables continuous adaptation of resources and delivery methods to reflect feedback from both learners and faculty. From a quality improvement perspective, this is essential as it can help to ensure the robustness of the activities and delivery methods.

### Planning the Evaluation

Evaluation planning must focus on the information you wish to gather and is linked to the originating rationale. For example, if you wish to learn more about learners' experiences of an SBE activity, then you may wish to create an evaluation form which focuses on provision of explanatory narrative detailing their experience. Alternatively, if you wish to measure satisfaction with various components of the SBE activity then you may wish to provide a questionnaire with indicators of levels of satisfaction to select from.

Firstly, it is important to recognise that there are a number of models available to assist you in structuring an evaluation of SBE. However, in this instance, the Kirkpatrick model will be considered as this is a recognised model which is frequently used for evaluating and measuring the impact of SBE (Allen et al., 2022). This is founded on four levels (Kirkpatrick, 1959):

- Level 1: Reaction – 'The degree to which participants find the training favourable, engaging, and relevant to their jobs'. Applying this to SBE could measure the learner's level of satisfaction with the SBE activity.
- Level 2: Learning and attitude – 'The degree to which participants acquire the intended knowledge, skills, attitude, confidence, and commitment based on their participation in the training'. Within the context of SBE, this could measure levels of knowledge attained and any changes in the learner's attitude.
- Level 3: Behaviour – 'The degree to which participants apply what they learned during training when they are back on the job'. As a consequence of an SBE activity, this could measure change in the learners' behaviour in their practice.
- Level 4: Outcomes or results – 'The degree to which targeted outcomes occur as a result of training, support and accountability package'. Within the modality of SBE, this could measure the learner's outcomes against a pre-determined criteria, for example, skills competency.

Whilst this has been adapted for the health and care environment and adopted by simulation-based educators for a number of years, this model was originally designed to help sales managers inform sales training and, as a consequence, improve financial outcomes for organisations (Yardley and Dornan, 2012). Despite implementation of this model for SBE evaluation, it is pertinent to note, however, that evaluation of this nature normally focuses on levels 1 and 2 of the model (Yardley and Dornan, 2012). Use of levels 3 and 4 are rare, as it is challenging to measure a change in behaviour or outcome after only one SBE activity (Kiegaldie et al., 2019). Furthermore this requires a collaborative approach to accomplish.

These four levels were determined in the seminal work of Kirkpatrick (1959). However, more recently in 2010, the focus of Kirkpatrick's model was updated to 'The New World Kirkpatrick Model', the aim being to maximise the transfer of learning to behaviour and subsequent organisational results. The rationale for this change was to better enable demonstration of the value of training to the organisation (Kirkpatrick and Kirkpatrick, 2010). The more contemporary model maintains the original four levels; however, there is the addition of new elements to each level to ensure that the model can be used and applied more effectively overall. Figure 9.1 details the components of the new world model (Kirkpatrick and Kyser-Kirkpatrick, 2010). When considering Fig. 9.1, note that the third and fourth levels continue to measure the changes in behaviour, and the impact of the effectiveness of the education, with perhaps more emphasis on the value it has provided to the organisation. Therefore, if starting the evaluation process at level 4, the focus would now be on what is most important for the organisation,

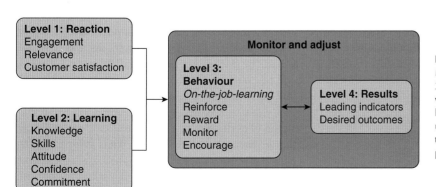

**Fig. 9.1** ■ Kirkpatrick's New World Model. (Kirkpatrick J, Kirkpatrick K. 2010 An Introduction to the New world Kirkpatrick model https://www.kirkpatrickpartners.com/wp-content/uploads/2021/11/Introduction-to-the-Kirkpatrick-New-World-Model.pdf accessed 16/08/22.)

rather than evaluation of learners' engagement and knowledge, as would be the focus in levels 1 and 2.

Although limited, there have been studies which explore the higher end of The New World Kirkpatrick model (Kirkpatrick and Kayser-Kirkpatrick, 2010) such as the impact of an educational intervention on patient outcomes through the use of simulation. An example of this may be laparoscopic surgery and bronchoscopy SBE, which also includes the use of deliberate practice (McGaghie et al., 2011a) which, they argue, can transfer directly to patient outcomes. Deliberate practice is purposeful, systematic, and highly structured with the aim of improving performance. It embodies consistent educational interventions and requires focussed attention (McGaghie et al., 2011b). This is pertinent because it is an example of a situation when levels 3 and 4 of Kirkpatrick's model of evaluation could be applied.

Planning SBE evaluation is an important element of the learning experience. Facilitators of SBE should consider 'did the session meet the intended learning objectives (ILOs)?' and 'was the SBE a good educational experience for learners?' Determining the answer to these questions requires collection of information from learners, and potentially faculty. The most common example of a data collection tool is a questionnaire – this can be distributed post-SBE or, alternatively, pre and post-SBE, depending on whether or not you wish to compare expectations to actual experience. Likert scales (Likert, 1932) are a useful way of gathering numerically scaled feedback from learners (Joshi et al., 2015). This feedback can support improvements moving forward as, depending on the structure of the Likert scales included, it can provide detail around level of satisfaction or dissatisfaction with components of the SBE activity. Traditionally Likert scales present choices aligned with the concepts of strongly disagree to strongly agree, with levels of agreement in between. It also advisable to include a neutral option.

The use of pre and post-questionnaires to evaluate a new educational course is demonstrated in Case Study 9.1.

## THE EVALUATION PROCESS

It is useful to evaluate all aspects of the SBE experience. This could therefore include seeking learner feedback regarding the pre-SBE resources and activities, SBE activity content and delivery, and post-SBE debriefing content and delivery. As part of this it may also be useful to evaluate the learner's perception of impact on practice moving forward as a consequence of the learning and SBE experience.

Moving forward with the evaluation process will involve revisiting the SBE activity plan, resources, and ILOs to ensure there is clarity around what it is that you wish to evaluate. It is also useful to involve faculty who will participate in the delivery of the SBE activity as they may have useful insights that they can share. If pre and post-session questionnaires are the option of choice, it is important to ensure that the questions presented to learners in both questionnaires are identical. The only difference should be that the pre-session questionnaire will focus on what learners expect, whereas the post-session questionnaire will require learners to share what they actually experienced and achieved. If, however, opting for a post-SBE activity evaluation only, then the questions will focus on gaining feedback after the SBE has taken place and will seek to gather information about the learning experience and knowledge gained.

Informing learners about the evaluation process is crucial for all of the reasons discussed as part of the context section of this chapter. The SBE environment should be safe and welcoming for learners and it is important to ensure that they are fully informed about any plans for evaluation of their learning experience. It is also important to ensure that they have freedom to consent to participate – or not – without any repercussions. Similarly, it is important to take steps to provide privacy for completion of evaluation documentation and to ensure that learners are aware that they should refrain from including any personal identifiers; this will help to protect anonymity for learners as part of the analysis process. In terms of confidentiality, learners should be reassured that their opinions and feedback will not be traceable to any one individual and, instead, will be considered as a collective for improvement of SBE activities and resources in the future. Alongside this, you may be considering dissemination and publication of evaluation findings. It is important to ensure that learners are aware of these plans prior to taking part in any aspect of the evaluation. It is also advisable to seek the consent of learners if wishing to publish and disseminate as this may be required if submitting an abstract for a conference or a scholarly publication. Evaluation data should be stored safely and securely in a locked drawer in a locked office or, alternatively if collected electronically, it should be stored on a secure password protected server in keeping with the data protection (Data Protection Act, 2018) requirements of your organisation.

The following evaluation case studies provide worked examples of using Likert scales pre and post-questionnaire.

## Evaluation Case Studies

Now that evaluation has been considered generally, two evaluation case studies are provided below to help contextualise your learning.

---

### CASE STUDY 9.1

#### BACKGROUND

During the pandemic, strain on hospitals and the reduction of staff permitted into the operating theatres meant that opportunities for paramedics, who are required to develop advanced airway management skills, were greatly reduced. However, to meet the requirements for programme completion, it was necessary to assess and determine their level of skill competence. In response to, and to meet the shortfall in theatre placements, an SBE study day was designed and delivered to the cohort of 46 paramedics. The skill of endotracheal intubation for paramedics is often only performed in a cardiac arrest situation. Therefore, one of the intended learning objectives (ILOs) from the SBE activities focused on clinical decision making in relation to airway management in the pre-hospital setting. The purpose of this was to support development of airway management skills and the consolidation of this knowledge through scenarios designed for their clinical settings and practice. This is important as the Stepwise Approach (Fig. 9.2) focuses on the application of an algorithm which directs the learner to use a structured approach to airway management (Soar et al., 2021).

The SBE study day incorporated several components including:
- On-line pre-learning
- Facilitated discussion on the day – including briefing and debriefing
- Practical workshops using high-fidelity manikins, with the ability to replicate difficult airway situations
- Scenarios which replicated pre-hospital settings to enable application of the skills in real-life situations

#### INFORMATION GATHERING FOR EVALUATION

All learners were issued with a pre and post-study day questionnaire, which they completed at the beginning and end of the day, respectively. The questions on each were identical, with the inclusion of an option for free text as part of the post-study day questionnaire. Figure 9.3 provides an overview of a segment of the latter, demonstrating the application of a 5-point Likert scale and the option of free text responses.

#### EVALUATION OUTCOMES

Learner evaluations were reviewed after the delivery of each study day and feedback regarding SBE content, omissions, or learner experience was addressed as appropriate following review and discussion with SBE faculty. Learner evaluations indicated that the SBE activities had enabled learners to achieve the ILOs. Learners also reported an increase in knowledge and skills for advanced and difficult airway management and non-technical skills, including clinical decision making, when comparing pre and post-study day questionnaire responses. In addition, with the exception of one learner, there was overall agreement that the scenarios assisted in consolidating knowledge and skills, as well as application of this to clinical practice (Fig. 9.4).

This evaluation provided some insight into learners' perception of their experience and learning. However, if wishing to measure the actual impact of the SBE activities on their real-life airway management skills, it would be necessary to conduct a longitudinal evaluation or research study. This can be challenging in the clinical setting.

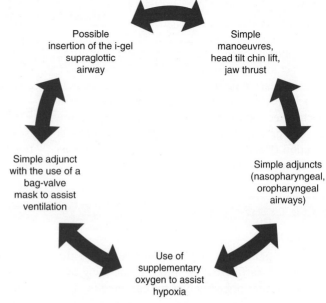

**Fig. 9.2** ■ The stepwise approach to airway management. (Morse J, Brown C, Morrison I, Wood C. 2019. Interprofessional learning in immediate life support training does effect TEAM performance during simulated resuscitation BMJ Simul Tecnol Enhanc Learn 19:5(4): 204-209.)

| We would also like your specific feedback on today's course | | | | |
| --- | --- | --- | --- | --- |
| The online learning improved your understanding of: | | | | |
| | Strongly agree | Agree | No opinion | Disagree |
| Drugs administration | ⬭ | ⬭ | ⬭ | ⬭ |
| Fluid administration | ⬭ | ⬭ | ⬭ | ⬭ |
| Resuscitation algorithms | ⬭ | ⬭ | ⬭ | ⬭ |
| | | | | |
| The workshops improved your knowledge and skills: | | | | |
| | Strongly agree | Agree | No opinion | Disagree |
| Stepwise approach to airway management | ⬭ | ⬭ | ⬭ | ⬭ |
| Intravenous cannulation and intraosseous insertion | ⬭ | ⬭ | ⬭ | ⬭ |
| Endotracheal intubation | ⬭ | ⬭ | ⬭ | ⬭ |
| | | | | |
| | Strongly agree | Agree | No opinion | Disagree |
| The scenarios helped in consolidating the knowledge into clinical practice | ⬭ | ⬭ | ⬭ | ⬭ |
| | | | | |
| Which parts of the course did you enjoy the most? | | | | |
| Were there any parts of the course you did not enjoy? | | | | |
| Is there any content you feel was not included today that would benefit future courses? | | | | |

SAS Dip HE: Practice Placement Adjustment Package (Post-course V1.2)

**Fig. 9.3** ■ An example of application of a Likert scale with free text options.

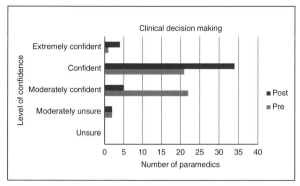
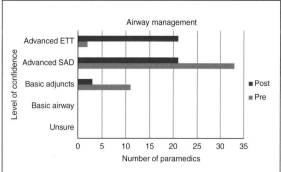
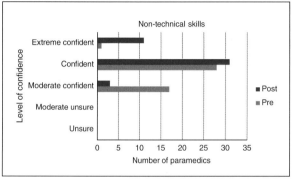
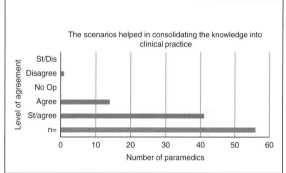

**Fig. 9.4** ■ Comparison evaluation of pre and post-study day feedback.

## CASE STUDY 9.2

### BACKGROUND

During the COVID-19 pandemic in 2020, the Scottish Nightingale Hospital was used as a simulation training centre, known as the National Skills Education Hub (NSEH), an interim base for clinical and SBE.

The aim of the NSEH was to ensure that essential education and training for health and care professionals continued despite the ongoing pandemic.

### GATHERING OF INFORMATION FOR EVALUATION

For evaluation purposes, a survey questionnaire (using Likert rating-scales) was developed and administered electronically (Ferguson, 2022) to health and care professionals who attended SBE at the NSEH. Data was collected relating to the physical learning space, personal safety, and the learning environment. Free text questions relating to what was reportedly learned during SBE activities were also included. A focus group was carried out with stakeholders, and facilitators took part in one-to-one telephone interviews. Two main themes emerged from the focus groups and telephone interviews.

### EVALUATION OUTCOMES

1. The size of the space allowed for social distancing while delivering SBE activities to larger groups than would have been possible in other venues. The flexibility of the space also allowed for delivery of education and training by multiple methods (such as structured theory lessons, practical teaching, and SBE).

2. Having all the resources and SBE activities concentrated in one building was deemed as positive by many of the facilitators and stakeholders because it enabled interprofessional working and provided easier access to support staff and resources.

These evaluation outcomes suggest that a centralised hub for SBE enabled NHS staff education and training to continue during the COVID-19 pandemic. The hub was evaluated positively in terms of personal safety, with the majority agreeing that they felt safe in the learning pods, had sufficient personal protective equipment and hand gel and that social distancing measures were adhered to. The larger space also ensured that multiple education and training activities could be delivered simultaneously, enabling interprofessional working.

## SIMULATION-BASED EDUCATION AND RESEARCH

The next part of this chapter will consider research in the context of SBE. However, the focus of this section will be a broad outline of the development of an SBE research project, with some hints and tips to get you started. It is important, however, to note that this will not include in-depth instruction on the research process itself. Should you wish to develop a more in-depth understanding about this, it is advisable to explore relevant research literature and evidence to ensure a well-informed approach for your research project.

### Rationale for Research

Health and social care education spanning all professions aims to equip both individuals and teams with the attributes, skills, and knowledge required to provide high-quality patient care (Ker, 2012). It has already been established that, to assess the impact of SBE, it is necessary to either evaluate or conduct research to demonstrate that the educational interventions are effective. The rationale for SBE research therefore logically falls into three main categories which include to:

- Inform future SBE training activities
- Measure the impact on learners' clinical practice
- Measure the impact on patient care

### Planning the Research

Planning, designing, and facilitation of SBE research can be challenging. For example, a Cochrane systematic review (Reeves et al., 2013) articulated some of the challenges, which included the lack of a thorough design process in some of this research. As a consequence, this research may not provide the evidence required to demonstrate the impact of interprofessional education on either patient outcomes or changes in health and care practices if not robustly planned and implemented. Therefore, the importance of ensuring that the research is planned and designed rigorously to address the research aims and objectives cannot be underestimated. To achieve this there are some hints and tips to remember when starting out on the research design process:

- At the outset it is imperative to be clear about the ILOs of the SBE activity as this will help to guide your research aims and objectives.

- Before embarking on the development of research aims and objectives, however, it is important to conduct a literature review in the chosen area for the research. This will help to ensure that you understand what evidence already exists, as well as what your contribution will be if you decide to move forward with the project.
- Understanding the potential for your contribution is important as it may be that you wish to contextualise, or add to, the body of evidence that already exists. Alternatively, it may be that you choose to consider an alternative project to generate new evidence where there is a gap.
- When developing the research question, it is a good idea to consider using a validated framework to assist with this process. For example (Methley et al., 2014):
  - PICO (Population, Intervention, Comparison, Outcome)
  - PICOS (Population, Intervention, Comparison, Outcome, Study Design)
  - SPIDER (Sample, Phenomenon of Interest, Design, Evaluation, Research Type)
- If choosing a qualitative approach, it is important to be aware that the number of participants required may be decided as data collection unfolds, rather than be determined in advance. This is because, most often, data collection in qualitative studies requires continuing to seek new participants until no new information transpires.
- If choosing a quantitative or mixed methods approach, consider seeking the advice of a statistician; they can help to determine the number of participants required for your research and will also be able to guide you regarding study design and statistical software.
- Contact your local research ethics committee (REC) for advice in structuring your research proposal and associated documentation (e.g., participant information sheet, consent form).
- Gatekeeper access must be sought to ensure research participants can be accessed and invited to participate in the study.
- It may be useful to generate a Gantt chart (to ensure clarity around timelines for access to participants, data collection and analysis).

- Integral to each element are funding considerations and the implications of these in terms of conducting any research project.

## MEASURING IMPACT – APPLYING THE 3Ts ROAD MAP

Now that planning the research process has been considered more generally, it is useful to think about applying a particular research framework in the context of SBE. For the purposes of this chapter, this will be the '3Ts Road Map' (Dougherty and Conway, 2008, p. 2319). This road map progresses through three phases (T1, T2, T3), with each of these building on the other with the aim to continually improve the delivery of health and care patient outcomes (Table 9.2).

The first phase T1 (Translation 1) is the beginning of the health and care education research process and involves research activity which focuses on testing clinical efficacy. T1 research studies are outcome-focused and are designed with the aim of improving knowledge, skills, and professionalism for either individuals or teams. These studies normally take place in the educational, rather than clinical, setting (Issenberg et al., 2011). The second phase, T2, aims to produce evidence of the effectiveness of T1 interventions, that is, outcome-focused research regarding who benefits from the SBE interventions, and the effectiveness of the care provided as a result. The final phase, and often the most difficult to quantify, is T3. This phase focuses on testing the quality of care at the point of delivery and can include quality and cost of care, service redesign, and subsequent scaling and dissemination of tested interventions (Dougherty and Conway, 2008).

When applying the 3Ts road map to measure the impact of SBE, it is important to recognise that the SBE activity must have been designed in a way that enables application of this approach. This includes consideration of the ILOs, the design of the SBE activities, and an over-arching aim to improve knowledge and application of technical and non-technical skills. The SBE activities delivered in the educational setting should also enable deliberate practice to acquire skills, alongside timely performance feedback from faculty. Brazil (2017, p. 1) suggests that Translational Simulation is an applicable term for describing the use of '*simulation activities that are directly focused on improving healthcare processes and outcomes*'.

## A RESEARCH CASE STUDY

This is an example of a quantitative study by Morse et al. (2019) that generated statistically significant findings stemming from an interprofessional resuscitation training research study.

The research was a randomised and blinded collaborative study assessing performance in a simulated resuscitation scenario, following the delivery of either an interprofessional or uniprofessional Resuscitation Council UK Immediate Life Support (ILS) course. The primary aim of the study was to investigate if the delivery of an interprofessional immediate life support course to medical and nursing students had an effect on team performance in a simulated resuscitation situation.

Equal numbers of both professions in the final 'student resuscitation teams' were achieved, comprising of three nursing and three medical students in each team. A total of 48 nursing students and 48 medical students were recruited to the study overall, equalling 96 learners. (For a flow diagram of the cohort allocations please refer to Fig. 9.5.)

| TABLE 9.2 | | | |
|---|---|---|---|
| **Application of 3Ts Road Map to Simulation-Based Education** | | | |
| 3Ts Phase ➡ | | | |
| Simulation-Based Education Activity ⬇ | T1 | T2 | T3 |
| **Increased or improved** | Knowledge, skills, attitudes, and professionalism | Patient care practices | Patient outcomes |
| **Target** | Individuals and teams | Individuals and teams | Individuals and public health |
| **Setting** | Simulation facility | Clinical setting | Clinical and community |

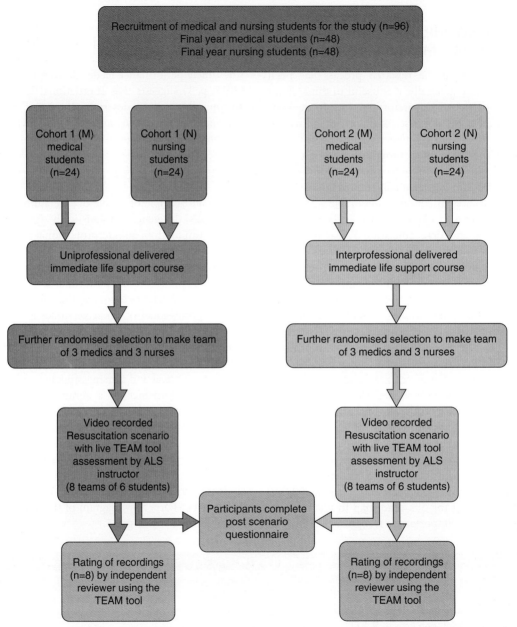

**Fig. 9.5** ■ A flow diagram showing the cohort allocations for an interprofessional resuscitation training study. *ALS,* Advance life support.

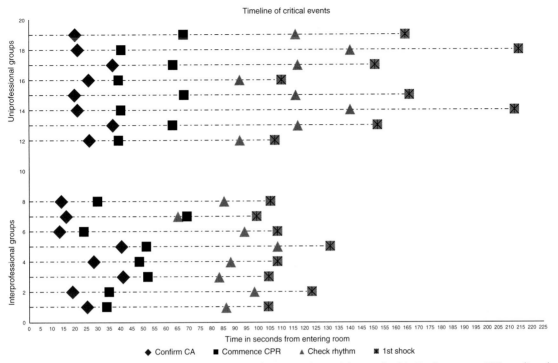

**Fig. 9.6** ■ Timeline of critical events for an interprofessional resuscitation training study. *CA,* Cardiac arrest; *CPR,* cardiopulmonary resuscitation.

Final year learners wishing to participate in this study would evaluate the teaching of ILS and would be randomly selected to participate in either the uniprofessional or the interprofessional courses.

Post intervention learners from both cohorts were allocated a time to attend the simulation suite and participate in a video recorded resuscitation scenario. Within each of the intervention-specific cohorts (inter-/uniprofessional), learners were further randomly assigned to form a 'resuscitation team' consisting of three medical and three nursing students. It was this randomisation, specifically to the uniprofessional cohort, that provided a baseline on which to measure the study's primary outcome, that the provision of an interprofessional ILS resuscitation course could lead to a change in team performance.

Each team of learners were asked to self-allocate their roles within the 'resuscitation team', including the team leader. In all but 3 of the 16 teams this was a medical student. To ensure consistency across all teams, the same scenario was used, aligned to the original ILS courses (a patient who deteriorates quickly into a ventricular fibrillation (VF) cardiac arrest and the need for timely defibrillation).

The video recordings from each of the resuscitation scenarios were reviewed by the researchers. Time-based outcomes (measured in seconds) from the team entering the room to starting an intervention were recorded and entered into the statistical software and appropriate testing applied. As the recordings had been taken using the Scotia Medical Observation and Training System (SMOTS) – a system for recording and playing back video, audio and, vital signs of a simulation – the accurate timings between these critical interventions were available on the video timeline. These time-recorded interventions, which were recorded and measured, included time from entry into room to confirming cardiac arrest, time to commencement of chest compressions, and time to delivery of first shock (Fig. 9.6).

This SBE study indicates that interprofessionally trained teams have significantly better time-based outcomes with regards to rhythm recognition and delivery of the first shock in a simulated cardiac arrest scenario. In clinical practice, in-hospital cardiac arrests are managed by interprofessional teams as opposed to uniprofessional groups; however, in the United Kingdom at undergraduate level, many of the mandatory life support courses continue to be delivered in a uniprofessional manner. This is despite increased regulatory emphasis on interprofessional team-based approaches to healthcare (Braithwaite et al., 2007).

Although assessment of team-based performance is vital, there are also many processes and task-based outcomes that, in clinical practice, have been shown to improve outcomes from cardiac arrest. Schneider et al. (1995), in their study involving a 'mobile intensive care unit' attending pre-hospital cardiac arrests found that process-related outcomes, time to intubation, and time to administration of adrenaline were significantly better following a standardised cardiac arrest training programme. However, what this study has added to the evidence base is that the interprofessionally trained teams performed pulse and rhythm check and defibrillation significantly quicker than the uniprofessionally trained teams. This, if transferred to clinical practice, would potentially influence patient outcomes for those experiencing cardiac arrest.

If this is the case, then it is possible to argue that this study moves the simulation based cardiac arrest educational literature up the scale of the New Model of Kirkpatrick's hierarchy of effectiveness to that of level 3 'behaviour'. Furthermore, it similarly moves this literature in the 3Ts model to T3. This demonstrates how an interprofessional learning simulation-based intervention can influence behaviour in clinical practice, and subsequent processes and measurements of team-based care during a post-test scenario.

Interprofessional education as a pedagogical approach to training has increased in recent years as educators now realise that healthcare occurs in teams and, to ensure effective training of teams, all members must learn together, emphasising the importance of this type of research.

## TOP TIPS

| Top Tip | Guidance |
| --- | --- |
| ■ **Understand evaluation and research in the context of simulation-based education (SBE)** | This is important as understanding will help to ensure that the correct approach is applied in the appropriate context. |
| ■ **Plan evaluation as part of planning the SBE activity** | This will help to ensure that the evaluation aligns to the intended learning objectives (ILOs). |
| ■ **Planning research is time-consuming and often requires advice from other experts** | It is a good idea to reach out to colleagues with research expertise, including your local research ethics committee. |
| ■ **Remember to check if ethics approval is required during the planning phase for both evaluation and research** | This will ensure that you adhere to requirements for both. |
| ■ **Honesty is the best policy!** | The aim should be to encourage authentic and frank feedback; it is important to ensure anonymity for both evaluation and research participants. |
| ■ **Practice makes perfect!** | Evaluation and research can be used to improve the creation and delivery of SBE activities. Accept that you may have to revisit and revise each time, depending on the outcome of each. |
| ■ **The ultimate aim is to improve care delivery** | Evaluation and research should also take account of the impact of SBE activities on care delivery. |

## SUMMARY

Health and social care education at all levels aims to equip aspiring professionals with the skills, knowledge, and attributes required to deliver safe, effective person-centred care. The primary aim of evaluation and research must be to ensure that learner preparedness is more effective, efficient, and economical, positively impacting on patient care. To this end, the goal of SBE evaluation and research is to demonstrate that SBE interventions are not only effective in the learning environment, but also transfer and translate into the clinical setting. The components and application of an evaluation and a research project have been considered as part of this chapter. As an SBE facilitator or faculty member it is important to consider which is most appropriate in what context, and to plan accordingly for your evaluation or research project. This will help to ensure that evidence is generated to add to, or augment, the body of SBE evaluation and research which already exists.

## REFERENCES

Abildgren, L., Lebahn-Hadidi, M., Mogensen, C.B., Toft, P., Nielsen, A.B., Frandsen, T.F., Steffensen, S.V., Hounsgaard, L., 2022. The effectiveness of improving healthcare teams' human factor skills using simulation-based training: a systematic review. Advances in Simulation 7 (1), 12.

Allen, L., Hay, M., Palermo, C., 2022. Evaluation in health professions education – Is measuring outcomes enough? Medical Education. 56, 127–136. https://onlinelibrary.wiley.com/doi/epdf/10.1111/medu.14654.

Braithwaite, J., Westbrook, J.I., Foxwell, A.R., Boyce, R., Devinney, T., Budge, M., et al., 2007. An action research protocol to strengthen system-wide inter-professional learning and practice [LP0775514]. BMC Health Services Research 7 (1), 1–10.

Brazil, V., 2017. Translational simulation: Not 'where?' but 'why?' A functional view of in situ simulation. Advances in Simulation 2 (1), 1–5.

Buljac-Samardzic, M., Doekhie, K.D., van Wijngaarden, J.D., 2020. Interventions to improve team effectiveness within health care: A systematic review of the past decade. Human Resources for Health 18 (1), 1–42.

Creswell, J.W., Creswell, J.D., 2017. Research Design: Qualitative, Quantitative, and Mixed Methods Approaches. Sage Publications.

Data Protection Act, 2018 [online]. Available at: Data protection: The Data Protection Act - GOV.UK (www.gov.uk). Accessed 9th October 2023.

Dougherty, D., Conway, P.H., 2008. The "3T's" road map to transform US health care: The "how" of high-quality care. JAMA 299, 2319–2321.

Ferguson, J., 2022. Evaluation of simulation training at the NHS Louisa Jordan Education Hub during COVID-19 – personal communication.

Gobbi, M., Monger, E., Weal, M.J., McDonald, J.W., Michaelides, D., De Roure, D., 2012. The challenges of developing and evaluating complex care scenarios using simulation in nursing education. Journal of Research in Nursing 17 (4), 329–345.

Issenberg, S.B., Ringsted, C., Østergaard, D., Dieckmann, P., 2011. Setting a research agenda for simulation-based healthcare education: A synthesis of the outcome from an Utstein style meeting. Simulation in Healthcare 6, 155–167.

Joshi, A., Kale, S., Chandel, S., Pal, D.K., 2015. Likert scale: Explored and explained. British Journal of Applied Science & Technology 7 (4), 396.

Ker, J., 2012. Review: The challenges of developing and evaluating complex care scenarios using simulation in nurse education. Journal of Research in Nursing 17 (4), 346–347.

Kiegaldie, D, Nestel, D, Pryor, E, Williams, C, Bowles, KA, Maloney, S & Haines, T, 2019. Design, delivery and evaluation of a simulation-based workshop for health professional students on falls prevention in acute care settings. Vol 6(3), pp. 1150–1162.

Kirkpatrick, J., 1959. Techniques for evaluation training programs. Journal of the American Society of Training Directors 13, 21–26.

Kirkpatrick, J., Kirkpatrick, K., 2010. An introduction to the New World Kirkpatrick model. https://www.kirkpatrickpartners.com/wp-content/uploads/2021/11/Introduction-to-the-Kirkpatrick-New-World-Model.pdf. Accessed 16/08/22.

Likert, R., 1932. A Technique for the Measurement of Attitudes. Archives of Psychology 22, 140.

Mathieson, C, 2007. What is the difference between research and evaluation? And why do we care? In N. L. Smith & P. Brandon (Eds.). Fundamental issues in evaluation. New York: Guilford Publishers.

McGaghie, W.C., Issenberg, S.B., Cohen, E.R., Barsuk, J.H., Wayne, D.B., 2011a. Translational. educational research: A necessity for effective health-care improvement. Chest 142, 1097–1103 2012.

McGaghie, W.C., Issenberg, S.B., Cohen, E.R., Barsuk, J.H., Wayne, D.B., 2011b. Does simulation-based medical education with deliberate practice yield better results than traditional clinical education? A meta-analytic comparative review of the evidence. Academic Medicine. 86 (6), 706–711. https://www.ncbi.nlm.nih.gov/pmc/articles/PMC3102783/.

Methley, A.M., Campbell, S., Chew-Graham, C., McNally, R., Cheraghi-Sohi, S., 2014. PICO, PICOS and SPIDER: a comparison study of specificity and sensitivity in three search tools for qualitative systematic reviews. BMC health services research 14 (1), 1–10.

Morse, J., Brown, C., Morrison, I., Wood, C., 2019. Interprofessional learning in immediate life support training does effect TEAM performance during simulated resuscitation. BMJ Simulation & Technology Enhanced Learning 19 (4), 204–209 5.

Reeves, S., Perrier, L., Goldman, J., Freeth, D., Zwarenstein, M., 2013. Interprofessional education: Effects on professional practice and healthcare outcomes. Cochrane Database Syst Rev 2013 (3), CD002213. https://doi.org/10.1002/14651858.CD002213.pub3.

Schneider, T., Mauer, D., Diehl, P., Eberle, B., Dick, W., 1995. Does standardized mega-code training improve the quality of pre-hospital advanced cardiac life support (ACLS)? Resuscitation 29 (2), 129–134.

Soar, J., Deakin, C.D., Nolan, J.P., Perkins, G.D., Yeung, J., Couper, K., et al., 2021. Adult advanced life support guidelines. Retrieved from https://www.resus.org.uk/library/2021-resuscitation-guidelines/adult-advanced-life-support-guidelines.

Sterner, A., Nilsson, M.S., Eklund, A., 2023. The value of simulation-based education in developing preparedness for acute care situations: An interview study of new graduate nurses' perspectives. Nurse Education in Practice 67.

Twycross, A., Shorten, A., 2014. Service evaluation, audit and research: what is the difference? Evidence-based nursing 17 (3), 65–66.

University of Cambridge Centre for Learning and Teaching, 2023. *Research and Evaluation Ethics* [online]. Available at Research & Evaluation Ethics | Cambridge Centre for Teaching and Learning. Accessed 8th October 2023.

Yardley, S., Dornan, T., 2012. Kirkpatrick's levels and education 'evidence'. Medical Education 46 (1), 97–106. https://doi.org/10.1111/j.1365-2923.2011.04076.x. https://www.kirkpatrickpartners.com/wp-content/uploads/2021/11/Introduction-to-the-Kirkpatrick-New-World-Model.pdf. Accessed 16/08/22.

# GLOSSARY

**Adverse Event:** • A harmful situation with a negative outcome for a service user

**Airway Management Skills:** • The clinical skills required to open or optimise a person's airway. These skills range from basic, where a non-invasive approach is taken using manual manoeuvres, to more advanced techniques. Advanced techniques require specialist training, and involves the use of airway adjuncts and specialist medical equipment

**Anatomical Models:** • A three-dimensional representation of anatomy

**Augmented Reality:** • Integration of digital information with the user's environment in real time to create a realistic environment

**Blooms' Taxonomy:** • A framework with six hierarchical categories used by educators to structure learning

**Carers:** • A family member or paid/unpaid helper who regularly provides care

**Competency-Based Education:** • A framework for learning, teaching and assessment which focuses on the learner's ability to master a skill

**Consumables:** • Commodities that are required to support simulation-based education and contribute to the authenticity of the scenario

**Critical Incident:** • A sudden or unexpected incident or situation within the workplace with the potential to cause harm

**Deliberate Practice:** • A teaching and learning strategy which aims to systematically separate each component of a skill to enable mastery of learning

**Didactic:** • An approach to teaching that focuses on instruction and passive learning rather than facilitation and active learning

**Embedded Professional:** • A member of the faculty who is immersed in the simulation scenario, provides information, and performs clinical tasks as the scenario unfolds

**Experiential Learning:** • The process of learning through experience and often more informally defined as learning by doing and through reflection

**Faculty:** • A group of staff, which can include clinical, technical, administration and academic staff, who as a collective deliver simulation-based education

**Fiction Contract:** • An explicit agreement between educators and learners wherein learner engagement is dependent on both parties

**Flipped Classroom:** • A learning and teaching strategy which aims to support and encourage active learning with engagement with defined pre-class resources

**Haptics:** • The use of technology and resources to simulate a realistic sensory experience for learners

**Fidelity:** • The level of realism experienced as part of the simulation scenario, often categorised as low, medium or high fidelity

**Iatrogenic Harm:** • Relating to illness caused by medical examination or treatment

**Immersive Simulation:** • The creation of scenarios which enable learners to experience authentic situations in a safe learning environment

**In Situ Simulation:** • The practice of engaging with simulation in a clinical environment

**Intended Learning Objectives:** • The particular knowledge and skills that it is intended that the learner will acquire on completion of a learning activity

**Interactive Manikin:** • A model which, by design, replicates the anatomy and physiology of a human

**Inter-professional Learning:** • Where two or more professional groups come together to learn with and from each other

**Laboratory-Based Simulation Education:** • Simulation-based education which takes place in a purpose-built simulation environment

**Learning Outcome:** • Measurable statements which outline what skills and knowledge learners should be able to develop as a consequence of undertaking the simulation-based education experience

**Major Incident:** • A situation or event with the potential for serious consequences which requires the involvement or intervention of a number of emergency services

**Mixed Reality:** • Simulation-based learning which blends both virtual and augmented reality

**Moulage:** • The creation of mock injuries, through the application of cosmetics, to create an authentic simulation experience

**Non-Technical Skill Development:** • Simulation-based learning which enables the development of social, cognitive and behavioural skills to enhance teamwork

**Part Task Trainers:** • A model which is designed to replicate a particular part of anatomy

**Personal Protective Equipment:** • Equipment worn to minimise the risk of exposure to potential hazardous substances

**Practice Placement Providers:** • An organisation which provides an opportunity to learn in practice

**Peer Learning:** • Learning from and with other learners

**Professional Regulatory Bodies:** • Organisations with professional governance for specific health and care disciplines

**Simulated Patient:** • A person who enacts the role of a patient in a simulation scenario

**Mastery Learning:** • A focused approach to skill development which recognises the individuality of each learner and their ability to develop and safely deliver the skill

**Situational Awareness:** • An awareness of, and ability to respond to, a particular environment

**Skill Acquisition:** • A teaching and learning approach that enables the development and improvement of set skills

**Telecare:** • An approach to care in the community which enables the utilisation of technology and devices to promote safety in the home environment

**Uniprofessional:** • One professional group

**Virtual Reality:** • The creation of a simulated environment to enable sensory stimulus

# INDEX

Page numbers followed by "b" indicate boxes, "f" indicate figures, "t" indicate tables.